The New GP

Changing roles and the modern NHS

Edited by

Jamie Harrison

Rob Innes

and

Tim van Zwanenberg

Foreword by

Sir Denis Pereira Gray

Radcliffe Medical Press

Radcliffe Medical Press Ltd
18 Marcham Road, Abingdon, Oxon OX14 1AA

British Library Cataloguing in Publication Data

A catalogue record for this book is available from the British Library.

ISBN 1 85775 492 1

Contents

Foreword

At a time of New Labour and a New NHS, it is natural that a book should appear entitled *The New GP*.

Change breeds anxiety and the current changes proposed for the NHS are as radical as any that have gone before and follow hard on the heels of a whole series of changes already assimilated into NHS general practice.

Furthermore, these NHS changes are both strategic and tactical, so that it is hard to concentrate on both the broad vision and the mass of detailed changes, all occurring together. This book sets out to place the changes for general practice in context. Its appearance is timely, and it is a most helpful contribution.

One problem facing many general practices is the vast array of papers in which changes are proposed. They come from many different sources, including the government, local NHS organisations such as PCGs in England and their equivalents elsewhere, statutory bodies like the GMC, and professional organisations like the Royal College of General Practitioners. This book is particularly good in three ways: it pulls the proposed changes together, it sets them in context, and the text is presented in an easy-to-read style.

The authors are experienced in the NHS and have analysed numerous documents well. This text will be a practical way for many colleagues in primary care to see the main proposals for change within the covers of a single book.

Sir Denis Pereira Gray OBE FRCP FRCGP FFPHM FMedSci
November 2000

Preface

So who, or what, is the new GP?

It is our choices, Harry, that show what we truly are, far more than our abilities.

JK Rowling

In one sense, every generation of general practitioners has been the 'new GP', propelled into the present by the power of political directives and the growth of clinical priorities, all of which imply 'choices' at both governmental and individual level. Yet the recent changes to the organisation and accountability of healthcare provision by a 'New Labour' government ('New Labour: New NHS'), allied to an increasingly consumerist society, make the demands on today's GPs significantly more complex than those which were placed on their predecessors.

In addition, the young doctors of today think and act differently (the new generation – 'generation X'), and every GP, whether young or old, ultimately cannot help but be shaped and influenced by the contemporary scene, with its growing concerns and widespread pressures. It is therefore clear that the rapidly evolving role of the GP of today and tomorrow is of major interest, and not just to doctors – for governments, health service managers and patients also have a stake in the game. In the light of this broad scenario, it is worth speculating on how one could complete the sentence beginning 'The new GP is ...'.

A practitioner

One view of the new GP is that he or she (and statistically it is currently more likely to be 'she') is a technician with communication skills. Competence in performing evidence-based practice is allied with expertise in communication – the ability to make real conversation with patients, listening with empathy and speaking with clarity. This doctor demonstrates 'hands-on' effectiveness and technical excellence.

A prophet

However, the performance of medical tasks in isolation from the wider social context is never enough. The prophetic role requires individual courage and demands a willingness to challenge the status quo, warning of the risks of proposed 'political' interventions. In this sense the prophet does not so much predict the future as foresee the consequences of certain actions – not least when they affect the lives of patients – acting as advocate and providing a critique of 'health' interventions (or the lack of them).

A pundit

The word 'pundit' comes from the Hindu world and reflects learning in Sanskrit, philosophy, religion and jurisprudence. The pundit is a learned teacher – a pedagogue. The new GP will be broadly based in thinking and experience, and will need to be aware of legal matters in an era of litigation, informed in the new ethics of gene therapy and the human genome project, and confident as a teacher of the new generation of medical students who will increasingly learn their medicine in the community setting.

A professional

With modernisation there is increased pressure on professional identity and the maintenance of professional values. The drive to flexible work practices also blurs the boundary lines between professional groupings. Is this job now the remit of the doctor or the nurse? And how will GPs manage their revalidation and regular appraisals in a climate of questioning and confusion over professional licensing and fitness to practise?

A partner

Increasingly, partnership will be viewed as something that the new GP enters into with patients, primary care team members and health service organisations, rather than with other doctors in a traditional profit-sharing partnership model. Young GPs are sceptical about long-term commitments and wary of being caught in inflexible working arrangements. Teamworking will take on greater significance, and the doctor–patient encounter will increasingly be a 'meeting between experts'.

A Harry Potter

JK Rowling's young wizard makes moral decisions and poses moral questions – in actual practice and to living communities. His is a world of struggle, fear, frailty and the ultimate triumph of goodness. As a new GP, Harry would reject the application of mere healing techniques, choosing rather to explore the limits of human resources (both in individuals and within wider society) and to examine the propriety of human expectations.

Harry Potter also finds himself engaging in battles (which he would rather not fight), discovering friends and forging alliances (in addition to making enemies and irritating opponents). In all of this he is guided by the desire to fulfil his destiny and live by the highest tradition of his calling (in his case, as a wizard). Perhaps the new GP might say the same.

Jamie Harrison
Rob Innes
Tim van Zwanenberg
November 2000

List of contributors

Tina Ambury Primary Care Physician, North Manchester Hospital, Manchester, Salford and Trafford Health Action Zone

Jamie Harrison General Practitioner and Associate Director of Postgraduate GP Education, University of Newcastle

Rob Innes Vicar of Belmont and Part-Time Lecturer in Theology, University of Durham

Di Jelley General Practitioner and Educational Research Fellow, University of Newcastle

Kevin McKenna General Practitioner and Medical Director, *NHS Direct* North-East

Cath O'Halloran Lecturer in Medical Education, University of Newcastle

Sir Denis Pereira Gray Chairman, Academy of Medical Royal Colleges

Mike Pringle Professor of General Practice, University of Nottingham

Laura Stroud Chair, North Tyneside Community Health Council

Stephen Sylvester General Practitioner and GP Tutor, Teesside

George Taylor General Practitioner and Deputy Director of Postgraduate GP Education, University of Newcastle

Tim van Zwanenberg Professor of Postgraduate General Practice, University of Newcastle

About this book

The New GP seeks to explain how and why the healthcare policies of the New Labour government that was elected in 1997 have had, and will continue to have, a major impact on the lives of individual general medical practitioners in the UK. Under the umbrella term of 'modernisation', this programme of 'reform' seeks to bring about a process of national renewal. Its key thrust is that it will be 'new', and that it cannot be avoided.

Part 1

The first part (Chapters 1 to 4) sets the scene, putting the rest of the book into a wider historical, social and political context. What is general practice anyway and is the traditional role of the generalist under threat (Chapter 1)? Does the consumerism of contemporary society undermine or benefit the provision of healthcare (Chapter 2)? How do governments and practitioners work out what each expects from the other (Chapter 3)? And what, in fact, is New Labour all about (Chapter 4)?

Part 2

The second part (Chapters 5 to 10) forms the solid core of the book, engaging with six critical (and practical) features of the modernisation programme. Managing demand for healthcare is a major priority. The application of triage via *NHS Direct* and walk-in centres is a key plank in the government's strategy (Chapter 5). Equally, the medical work-force should be better equipped for the task of providing clinical services, through continuing professional development (Chapter 6) and appraisal (Chapter 7). Greater accountability of doctors, and with it quality improvement, will come from revalidation (Chapter 8) and clinical governance (Chapter 9). Finally, the human resource of the NHS will become more effective and efficient through flexible patterns of working (Chapter 10), within the context of the new primary care organisations – primary care groups and trusts.

Part 3

The third and final part of the book (Chapters 11 to 14) looks to the future. What do patients expect from their doctors and how can they participate in discussions about where the health service is going (Chapter 11)? What about the views of the younger doctors who are becoming GPs and could expect to work in general practice in the NHS for the next 20 to 30 years (Chapter 12)? And is there a way forward, which brings together the conflicting views and concerns of the various parties in the debate, resulting in a positive synthesis and hopeful collective outcome (Chapter 13)?

The reader must judge how he or she will work through the book, perhaps choosing to concentrate on the social and political rather than the practical, or vice versa. Whichever course of action is taken, critical engagement with the issues should prove a thought-provoking and stimulating task.

Acknowledgements

We are grateful for the support and help of a wide variety of people in producing this book. In particular, we would like to thank the contributors for their enthusiasm and hard work. Many colleagues, both young and more senior, have helped to clarify our thinking by challenging us and asking questions. A group of senior managers from health and social services, as well as clinicians, theologians and patients' representatives participated in a discussion with us on the new GP. They included Kevin McKenna, Phil Adams, Ruth Etchells, Claire Lazenby, Christina Edwards, Peter Hill, Di Jelley, Stephen Sylvester, Robert Song, Jane Macnaughton, Laura Stroud, Liz Jordan, Ken Jarrold and Robin Hudson. We thank them all for their thoughtful ideas and comments. We have, as ever, relied on our primary care team colleagues at Cheveley Park Medical Centre, Durham, and Collingwood Surgery, North Shields. They have made us think, and provided us with constant reminders of reality. Gillian Nineham from Radcliffe Medical Press has encouraged us throughout. Angela McLaughlin has worked efficiently and with great calm and good humour to produce the final typescript, and considerable thanks are due to her.

For Anne, Helen and Linda

PART 1

Setting the scene

CHAPTER ONE

So what is general practice?

Jamie Harrison

You see the advantage of always consulting me.

Mr Gibson (from *Wives and Daughters*)[1]

This opening chapter sets the scene for the rest of the book. How is general practice to be defined, and what are the issues behind talk of the new GP? Is it realistic for GPs to provide personal, primary and continuing medical care?

Introduction

We would all like to believe that the world benefits from our own specific contribution. This is especially true if we belong to one of the so-called caring professions, where the work we do is perceived by the rest of society as a communal 'good' – something which increases social cohesion. How shocking, then, when this notion of goodness is challenged by events such as those in Hyde in Greater Manchester, where the misuse of medical power by one doctor took away lives, subverted trust and inevitably undermined wider notions of professional standing and status.[2]

The standing and status of GPs have historically been linked to questions not only of their role in society but also of their clinical expertise. This latter element is expressed in terms of the extent to which a GP possesses a discrete body of specialist or specialised knowledge – that is, knowledge and insights not typically available to the general public, and specific to the profession of general practice. At a time when access to the Internet and call centres is making medical information available to all, this issue of 'specialised' knowledge is brought into sharper focus, leading GPs as a profession to ask fundamental questions about their purpose and role definition.

It may be asked whether it is the GP's *possession* of medical knowledge (however defined) or its *application* in day-to-day practice that sets him or her apart – from the public, from other primary care practitioners and from hospital doctors. There is also uncertainty about whether any attempt to define a discrete, individualistic, medical role is acceptable in the modernised pattern of contemporary healthcare, with its emphasis on flexibility, teamwork, skill mix and working to guidelines and protocols.

General practitioners appear by nature to be individualists who value their autonomy and the ability to work out their own destinies. They can be intolerant of what they perceive as interference, and resent being told what to do. However, the world outside is no longer willing to allow doctors to make their own rules. The profession itself is beginning to recognise this, but much still needs to be done to re-establish its professional self-understanding.[3]

Specialist or generalist?

Some definitions

Recent discussion in the *British Medical Journal* once again raised questions about how to define general practice.[4,5] In an effort to respond to the apparent unwillingness of some governments, and the European Commission, to improve postgraduate training for general practice, on the grounds that GPs were not 'specialists', a new definition of a general practitioner was offered (*see* Box 1.1).

Box 1.1:   A new definition of the general practitioner[3]

The general practitioner is a specialist trained to work in the front-line of a healthcare system and to take the initial steps to provide care for any health problem(s) that the patient may have. The general practitioner takes care of individuals in society, irrespective of the patient's type of disease or other personal and social characteristics, and organises the resources available in the healthcare system to the best advantage of the patient. The general practitioner engages with autonomous individuals across the fields of prevention, diagnosis, cure, care and palliation, using and integrating the sciences of biomedicine, medical psychology, and medical sociology.

The editorial asked whether this definition helped or hindered a proper understanding of general practice for today. The authors were clear that, at least in the English language, the terms 'generalist' and 'specialist' were opposites, and this created problems. They commented that, in many European countries, general practitioners have needed to claim specialist status in order to achieve recognition as a separate discipline. However, in the UK, this recognition has been achieved by exploiting the notion of opposites and showing that the expertise of the generalist is complementary to that of the specialist, and that the two are profoundly interdependent.[5]

The authors of the editorial went on to point out that the focus of general practice is broad and involves integrating the complexity of medical care in the patients' context – that ability to switch between different perspectives (e.g. biomedical, humanities) related to patients' health problems. This contrasted with the position of the traditional medical specialist, whose expertise is in grappling with the complexity of a defined and narrow biomedical area. Iona Heath has expressed well the particular challenge presented to the generalist:

> *All aspects of human existence are legitimate concerns of the general practitioner provided that they are presented as a problem by the patient. This means that the general practitioner is obliged to deal with the complexity of each individual patient and should never be content to respond to a patient by saying 'That's not my business or my problem.' Each person and each context is unique, and this is the joy and the challenge of general practitioner care.*[6]

In *The Paradox of Progress* we find James Willis agreeing with this perspective. He approaches the problem of the generalist by employing the idea that you can define generalists quite precisely not in terms of what they do, but in terms of what they do *not* do (*see* Box 1.2).

Box 1.2:   Willis' definition of a generalist[7]

A generalist never says that something is of no interest to him.

In this way Willis reinforces the open nature of general practice for him, as medicine without boundaries. The patient defines the problem.

Creating boundaries

Increasingly, however, general practitioners are trying to limit their remit and the extent of their personal responsibilities. Whether it is due to viewing themselves purely as supervisors of care packages, providers of only a limited range of medical interventions or working increasingly as managers within healthcare organisations, a redefinition of the GP role is taking place. This is allied to a reduction in their hours of availability to patients. A mismatch has developed between what is believed about GPs (the rhetoric) and what GPs actually do (the reality), as reflected in Box 1.3.

Box 1.3:   Rhetoric and reality in the GP role

	Rhetoric	*Reality*
• The GP provides:	a full range of services	limited services
• The GP works to:	a biopsychosocial model	a bio(psycho) model
• The GP is:	available at all hours	limited in availability

A full range of personal services?

A survey of the attitudes of GPs in Avon some years ago found that, in general, doctors agreed that their responsibilities for patient care included problems related to internal medicine (e.g. diabetes and hypertension). Less consensus was found in their responses to technical procedures (e.g. resection of ingrowing toenails), and to gynaecological, ortho-paedic and psychosocial problems. The authors of the survey concluded that general practitioners were gradually abandoning technical aspects of medicine to specialists, without defining a compensating role. They argued that, in the light of this trend, the responsibilities of general practitioners should be more clearly defined by the profession.[8]

In collaboration with Dutch colleagues, Michael Whitfield went on to conduct a comparison study seeking to determine whether this loss of technical involvement was specific to English general practitioners. The study's findings supported a general shift away from practical interventions, although this was less marked for Dutch GPs. However, the Avon GPs took more responsibility for chronic problems than did their continental counterparts.[9]

After the imposition of the 1990 Contract for general practitioners, sessional payments were introduced to try to encourage the performance of minor surgery, with similar inducements to take on structured health promotion and disease management. The latter clinics were later removed from the payment system, as they were felt to be unscientific.[10] It is worth noting that practice nurses and nurse practitioners have increasingly replaced GPs as the clinicians involved in well-woman, chronic disease management and health promotion clinics. What does this say about GPs and their work in dealing directly with those who suffer from chronic diseases?

A biopsychosocial model of healthcare?

Chris Dowrick and his colleagues have found that GPs themselves do not believe that they should be concerned with the full gamut of human experience – biological, psychological and social. The members of the Royal College of General Practitioners whom they surveyed believed that GPs should work to a bio(psycho) rather than a biopsychosocial model of healthcare.[11]

The idea that there is a mismatch between what society could reasonably expect of GPs and what GPs would consider legitimate is intriguing. For example, individuals with learning disabilities may receive satisfactory medical treatment but be denied regular health promotion activity and structured health checks, including assessment of hearing and eyesight. That apparently is the job of other services, not of GPs.[12]

Available all hours?

If the social aspects of a patient's problems, as well as certain technical interventions, are clearly beyond the remit of today's GPs, have general practitioners also abandoned any vestigial belief in the notion of the self-sacrificing GP available for 24 hours a day to his or her patients? But perhaps that was never quite what it seemed:

> *The character of the village family doctor who attended to his people as part of a vocation that embodies fatherly self-sacrifice is, to a significant extent, a nostalgic myth. People knew that you did not visit the doctor unless there was something seriously wrong. You might have to pay for treatment. And you could expect an irate response if he felt you were wasting his time.*[13]

The shift to out-of-hours GP co-operatives, the use of deputising services and the development of extended rotas suggest that GPs look to protect their time and limit their availability to patients. The increasing use of locums and salaried doctors within practices also reduces daytime opportunities for patients to see a personal doctor. In view of all this uncertainty, it is certainly worth re-visiting the professional role of the GP and the training that is required to fulfil it.

The future general practitioner

In 1972 the Royal College of General Practitioners (RCGP) published the book *The Future General Practitioner*.[14] This 266-page document, which was written by six of the College's 'wise men', followed two short reports which had set the scene for the newly emerging three-year vocational training programme, namely *The Educational Needs of the Future General Practitioner* (1969)[15] and *The Future General Practitioner. Problems of Organising his Training* (1971).[16]

The book set down the content of general practice for educational purposes, dividing this into five areas as outlined in the 1969 report (*see* Box 1.4). It made clear the fact that clinical medicine is not restricted to health and disease, and that during the consultation with the patient, the doctor will draw on all of the clinical practice areas equally.

Box 1.4:   The five areas of general practice for training purposes[15]

- Clinical practice – health and disease
- Clinical practice – human development
- Clinical practice – human behaviour
- Medicine and society
- The practice

The authors of *The Future General Practitioner* used the report of 1969 to define what a general practitioner actually did. They identified a job definition (*see* Box 1.5) which stated, as an ideal, the work to be done and the role to be played by the trainee on completing the (vocational training) programme.[14] They had high expectations that the programme of training would mould the doctors involved, leading them to *behave* in a way that was consistent with that ideal.

Box 1.5:   A concise definition of the general practitioner's job[14]

The general practitioner is a doctor who provides personal, primary and continuing medical care to individuals and families. He may attend his patients in their homes, in his consulting-room or sometimes in hospital. He accepts the responsibility for making an initial decision on every problem his patient may present to him, consulting with specialists when he thinks it appropriate to do so.

He will usually work in a group with other general practitioners, from premises that are built or modified for the purpose, with the help of paramedical colleagues, adequate secretarial staff and all the equipment which is necessary. Even if he is in single-handed practice, he will work in a team and delegate when necessary.

His diagnoses will be composed in physical, psychological and social terms. He will intervene educationally, preventively and therapeutically to promote his patient's health.

The problems with this model – the new GP

However, this ideal is now under scrutiny, not least with regard to what constitutes 'personal, primary and continuing medical care'. What do these notions mean today, and are the concepts behind them valued by doctors, patients and the government or health service funders?

Moreover, the world and its doctors have moved on. Not only is there a modernising agenda for the NHS, but the new GPs demand a 'do-able job' as well as a 'life outside medicine'. The job, as defined above, appears to allow neither of these. The College's 1969 definition has the remit of providing an ideal of the work to be done and the role to be played by the typical general practitioner. Yet there is no doubt that the idea of the traditional, constantly available personal doctor who provides comprehensive services is being seriously questioned, and by all of the parties in the discussion.

Do we still want personal doctors?

Put in its sharpest form, the question is whether today's patients would either want or expect 'my doctor'. Under the headline *Medics on Web force Dr Finlay to retire*,[17,18] a national broadsheet recently reflected on the publication of the BMA's discussion document *Shaping Tomorrow*.[19] The newspaper went on to assert that the age of AJ Cronin's archetypal GP Dr Finlay was over, and that patients now telephone nurses directly or seek help via the Internet, accepting the loss of personal relationships with doctors in return for speedier access to healthcare advice. In contrast, Sir Denis Pereira Gray offers the perspective quoted in Box 1.6.

Box 1.6:   The centrality of the personal relationship in general practice[19]

If I see one of my partner's patients, I reckon I am a quarter less effective. If I am covering for a neighbouring practice, I reckon I am a half less effective.

There's a trade-off between how long people are prepared to wait to see the doctors they want. Some wait a worryingly long time.

I think the people who don't experience human relations intensely in primary care over the years always devalue those relationships. It's difficult to convey the importance of that relationship if you haven't experienced it.

The intensity of the doctor–patient relationships is seen not only in the writings of AJ Cronin but also, for example, in Elizabeth Gaskell's *Wives and Daughters*,[1] where the local doctor, Mr Gibson, forms deep and complex connections with his patients – much to his new (second) wife's displeasure when she feels excluded. At one point, he challenges her over a breach in confidentiality – she has been eavesdropping (*see* Box 1.7).

Box 1.7:   A conversation from *Wives and Daughters*[1]

Mr Gibson: *Don't you know that all professional conversations are confidential? That it would be the most dishonourable thing possible for me to betray secrets which I learn in the exercise of my profession?*

Mrs Gibson: *Yes, of course.*

Mr Gibson: *Well! And are not you and I one in these respects? You cannot do a dishonourable act without my being inculpated in the disgrace. If it would be a deep disgrace for me to betray a professional secret, what would it be for me to trade on that knowledge?*

He was trying hard to be patient, but the offence was of that class which galled him insupportably.

Is that high sense of duty and responsibility towards individual patients, as evidenced by fictional doctors such as Dr Finlay and Mr Gibson, highly valued by patients today? The picture is complex. Richard Baker's 1996 study of patient satisfaction with their consultations found that satisfaction declined where list sizes were increasing, if a personal list system was absent, and if the practice was a training practice (i.e. patients were expected to see trainees). He concluded that provision of a personal service enhanced patient satisfaction. In his view, general practitioners need to review the organisation of their practices to ensure an acceptable balance between the requirements of modern clinical care and the wishes of patients.[20]

Continuity of care – myth or reality?

However, back in 1981, Cartwright and Anderson pointed out that over one-third of patients attending a surgery were prepared to see another doctor straight away rather than wait only half an hour to see their own doctor.[21] How much were they valuing the experience of continuity of care in practice?

George Freeman has studied this issue from the perspective of both the doctor and the patient. A recent paper makes some key points (*see* Box 1.8).

Box 1.8: Key points on continuity of care in general practice[22]

- Changes in society and professional developments are squeezing out traditional continuity of care.
- Patients want doctors who listen and solve problems more than they want longitudinal continuity.
- Longitudinal continuity should be replaced by personal continuity, where medical decisions are taken by the patient in consultation with the doctor.
- Seeing the same patients increases job satisfaction and education, but requires a high level of personal commitment.
- A policy of personal continuity requires commitment from all members of the primary care team.
- Continuity of care with the whole team may be more feasible than continuity with one doctor.

Chris Dowrick believes that significant change has occurred in the way in which GPs perceive what they are actually doing in the consultation:

I believe that there is a subtle but distinct shift currently taking place in the way in which GPs describe their encounters with patients. From considering them in terms of the quality of the relationship, we are now more likely to discuss them in terms of good or poor communication. This change may in part reflect increasing expertise and professionalisation among GPs. However, I suggest that it is also a consequence of the contextual differences in general practice ... principally the reduction in continuity of care.[23]

Conclusion

The RCGP definition of a GP's job includes within it the tension of how to provide personal, primary and continuing medical care whilst at the same time maintaining personal expertise, health and fitness to practise. The definition centres on the individual, but also encourages group practice and appropriate delegation to others. It is perhaps this latter aspect which most troubles GPs of today. Are they to seek to sustain *breadth* (offering wide-ranging personal services and availability to patients) or to develop *depth* (with sub-specialisation, limited availability and a designated place in the practice team)?

With increasing consumerism and governmental monitoring comes the overwhelming pressure to tailor services to external expectations – of speed of access, quality of information and effectiveness of action. Here the GP faces the challenge of the emerging primary care organisations, where new ways of working collaboratively with a variety of colleagues, and an openness to new technologies, appear to offer the way ahead. We can be left wondering what remains at the heart of general practice. Indeed, the question for the new GP might be 'Can the generalist survive?'.

Summary points

- Historically, GPs' standing has been linked with their role in society as well as their medical expertise.
- There has been a debate in Europe about whether a GP is a specialist.
- In the UK, the GP has been seen as a generalist both complementary to the specialist and interdependent with them.
- In recent years, GPs have started to create boundaries to their role, limiting their availability and the services they offer.
- The model of a generalist providing 'personal, primary and continuing medical care' is under scrutiny.
- In particular, personal doctoring and continuity of care are being challenged as mere rhetoric.
- Increasing consumerism and government monitoring exert pressure to tailor services to external expectations.
- New ways of working collaboratively with a variety of colleagues and an openness to new technologies may be the way ahead, but can the generalist survive?

References

1 Gaskell E (1866) *Wives and Daughters.* Penguin Books, Harmondsworth.

2 This refers to the case of Harold Shipman, a general practitioner in Greater Manchester, who in January 2000 was convicted of murdering a number of his patients.

3 Irvine D (1999) The performance of doctors: the new professionalism. *Lancet.* **353**: 1174–7.

4 Olesen F, Dickinson L and Hjortdahl P (2000) General practice – time for a new definition. *BMJ.* **320**: 354–7.

5 Heath I, Evans P and van Weel C (2000) The specialist of the discipline of general practice. *BMJ.* **320**: 326.

6 Heath I (1995) *The Mystery of General Practice.* The Nuffield Provincial Hospitals Trust, London.

7 Willis J (1995) *The Paradox of Progress.* Radcliffe Medical Press, Oxford.

8 Whitfield M and Bucks R (1988) General practitioners' responsibilities to their patients. *BMJ.* **297**: 398–400.

9   Whitfield M, Grol R and Mokkink H (1989) General practitioners' opinions about their responsibility for medical tasks: comparison between England and The Netherlands. *Fam Pract.* **6**: 274–8.

10 van Zwanenberg T (1998) Strategic shifts. In: J Harrison and T van Zwanenberg (eds) *GP Tomorrow.* Radcliffe Medical Press, Oxford.

11 Dowrick C, May C, Richardson M *et al.* (1996) The biopsychosocial model of general practice: rhetoric or reality? *Br J Gen Pract.* **46**: 105–7.

12 Kerr M, Dunstan F and Thapar A (1996) Attitudes of general practitioners to caring for people with learning disabilities. *Br J Gen Pract.* **46**: 92–4.

13 Harrison J and Innes R (1997) *Medical Vocation and Generation X.* Grove Books, Cambridge.

14 Royal College of General Practitioners (1972) *The Future General Practitioner.* Royal College of General Practitioners, London.

15 Royal College of General Practitioners (1969) The educational needs of the future general practitioner. *J R Coll Gen Pract.* **18**: 358–60.

16 Royal College of General Practitioners (1971) *The Future General Practitioner. Part 1. Problems of Organising his Training. Report from General Practice 14.* Royal College of General Practitioners, London.

17 Cronin AJ (1978) *Dr Finlay of Tannochbrae.* New English Library, London.

18 Millward D (2000) Medics on Web force Dr Finlay to retire. *The Daily Telegraph,* 23 February.

19 Mihill C (2000) *Shaping Tomorrow: Issues Facing General Practice in the New Millennium.* BMA, London.

20 Baker R (1996) Characteristics of practices, general practitioners and patients related to levels of patients' satisfaction with consultations. *Br J Gen Pract.* **46**: 601–5.

21 Cartwright A and Anderson R (1981) *General Practice Revisited.* Tavistock Press, London.

22 Freeman G and Hjortdahl P (1997) What future for continuity of care in general practice? *BMJ.* **314**: 1870–3.

23 Dowrick C (1997) Rethinking the doctor–patient relationship in general practice. *Health Soc Care Commun.* **5**: 1–4.

CHAPTER TWO

The world in which we live

Jamie Harrison

The more you have, the more you want.

Anon.

This chapter lays out four models of society for today. Are we to be part of a burgeoning consumer society dominated by rapid communication, or is it possible to discover better ways of relating to one another? And can doctors avoid being overwhelmed by the needs of others?

Introduction

Wherever you stop to look – in a popular GP weekly periodical, in the health or economics column of a broadsheet newspaper, or even in the editorial of a reputable medical journal – the consensus is clear. We are experiencing a consumerist boom, or at least a boom in consumer expectations.

Within the Western market economies, the demand for both good health and high-quality healthcare services is rising exponentially. Governments and other funders struggle to manage demand and to balance the budgets. The implications of rising expectations for 'health' and 'healthcare', and the pressures generated by new understandings of what it might mean to be healthy, are worrying. 'Healthy' risks being equated with 'happy', and the desire to have health is confused with a pain-free existence. The 'very best' level of care is only just 'good enough'.[1]

In all of this there remains a fundamental question. Must we learn to accept the dominant consumerism, with its vision of a future that can only become more out of control and more free-market driven? Or is there an alternative possibility, or collection of possibilities, that can alter the shape of thinking and taking action in this area?

Box 2.1:   Four models of society

- The consumer society
- The call society
- The service society
- The covenant society

The consumer society
Consumerism as a way of life

Consumerism is at the heart of modern life. Yet it is worth remembering that, even as long ago as the eighteenth century, material possessions had begun to be valued less and less for their durability and more and more for their fashionableness.

Increasingly we find that each day is shaped by our individual patterns of consumption – how, why and what we consume – in terms of both goods and services. Even the act of daily exercise takes on the need for a private gym and the designated designer footwear. For many, consumerism itself masquerades as the new religion, replacing the other failed -*isms* of our generation, a process that is aided and abetted by the loss of nerve of the traditional political parties, the collapse of communism and the self-parodying of postmodernism. Descartes' 'I think therefore I am' gives way to the consumer's 'I shop therefore I am'.

Steven Miles reflects this theme in the title of his book *Consumerism – as a Way of Life*. For Miles:

> *Everyday life in the developed world appears, at least at a common-sense level, to be dominated by our relationship with consumer goods. Wherever we go, whether in the High Street, the museum, the airport, the sports stadium, the doctor's surgery or our very own living-room, consumerism is touted as the answer to all our problems, an escape from the mundane realities of everyday life.*[2]

Early on in the book Miles makes it clear that his task is to ask to what extent individuals and societies are in control of their relationship with the consumption of such goods. Who, if you like, is in charge? Who is the master or mistress? Who is the servant or slave?

Whether consumerism itself would claim such a broad remit as to be the 'answer to all our problems' is debatable. What is clear, however, is that 'consumerism' *per se* cannot be treated as some isolated or abstract concept that is separate from the real world.

Consumerism lives and breathes within actual social contexts, and it is found in the everyday experience of individuals. Their expectations both fuel and critique the consumerist world which we all inhabit.

What then does a consumerist society look and feel like? Is it exclusively a place of self-gratification, *'excessively preoccupied with consumption'* (to borrow a phrase from Yiannis Gabriel and Tim Lang[3])? Defining consumerism in such a pejorative way suggests a self-oriented, hedonistic view of the art of consuming. However, Steven Miles prefers to describe the social impact of consumerism as ubiquitous rather than excessive:

> *Consumer goods and services appear to surround us, but need not necessarily be a negative influence on our lives. As such, consumerism should not and cannot be morally condemned, but must rather be considered in a systematic fashion as an arena within which social lives are currently constructed.*[2]

If Miles is unwilling at this point to dismiss consumerism as morally corrupt (and corrupting), his text is ultimately a critical one, leaving the reader to make up their own mind about the social and ideological impact of consumerism. What is clear is that two of the foundational tenets of consumerism, namely choice (for the consumer) and democratisation (to include everyone), struggle when faced by the challenge of public services such as the NHS:

> *The problem here is that politicians have found it very hard to sustain a high-quality public sector which incorporates adequate welfare provision, in a system in which consumerism is intended to provide all the answers.*[2]

The consuming paradox

The experience of consuming can be analysed from a number of different perspectives. At one level it is about transactions between vendors and customers. There are economic aspects, not least concerning how money is raised to pay for the goods and services received, as well as the financial implications of employing staff to provide the goods and services that are on offer.

Perhaps more interesting is the perspective of what the act of consuming actually 'does' to the people concerned. How, if you like, should the 'consuming experience' be categorised? For many, the act of consuming appears fascinating, arguably fulfilling and personally appealing. Yet the requirement to keep on consuming, with its complex programme of self-generating activities, itself becomes a dominant, controlling influence. The consumer is both trapped and free at the same time, caught in what might be termed the 'consuming paradox'.

Where consumption begins to play an increasingly important role in people's everyday lives, where people are offered not only what they need but also what they desire, 'wants' actively become 'needs'. Miles quotes the example of spectacles. Previously, a very basic, functional pair of spectacles might have been sufficient for the partially sighted customer. Now, in a consumer culture, functional items become designer items, and a pair of spectacles becomes another means by which individuals can express their self-identity.

Of course, many things that started life as wants rightly become needs in a civilised society. Analgesia in childbirth, parents staying overnight with their sick children, and patient access to medical records are now seen as proper, routine ways of doing things. Yet the message is clear if we believe the old proverb that 'the more you have, the more you want'.

Consumerism and health

Whether or not we have a right to be healthy,[1] there is no doubt that, in the UK, our ideology of consumerism demands that individuals have the right to ready access to healthcare. At present, this right also assumes that access should be at no cost (i.e. 'free') at the point of service provision, with health service funding provided through direct taxation. This continues to be clear government policy.

Such 'rights' have been formalised in government-initiated charters, notably the Patients' Charter in the case of healthcare. Charters bring with them consumer rights but not necessarily consumer responsibilities. We have argued that the concept of citizenship calls for real mutuality, where both parties in the relationship are actively engaged together, rather than one party (the consumer) being passive and the other (the service provider) remaining under an imposed obligation.[1] Where citizens and healthcare professionals interact well, an experience that differs markedly from that of consumer–provider results (*see* Box 2:2).

Box 2.2:   Good citizen–professional interactions[1]

Such interactions:

* manifest consistent technical soundness
* engage the whole human experience
* recognise the citizen as a person with unique identity and responsibility
* use resources appropriately
* lead to mutually acceptable outcomes
* help to improve the health of individuals and populations
* are realistic and affirming
* share responsibility and decision making.

If, then, the consumer model of society is inadequate, is its current extension into a 'call society' even more of a problem?

The call society

In the call society we are faced by the urgent command that cannot be ignored, the directive that must be answered, the summons that will not wait. This is the world of instant action and response. Even just a few years ago it was possible to receive a letter in the morning post, mull over its contents for a day or so, formulate a reply, get that typed and then return the response via the postal delivery service. All in all, the process from start to finish lasted about four days. How different the world is now, where leaving the response to a fax, email or telephone message for a mere four hours is considered either unacceptable or just downright difficult to do.

Increasingly we live in what might be termed 'the call culture', where time is precious and every question needs an immediate reply. Instant accessibility has replaced reasonable availability. Just count the number of people you pass in the street speaking into their mobile phones. Even sitting quietly on a train reading a book is no longer regarded as an acceptable relaxation from the stresses of modern life.

This potentially dehumanising, call-dominated society places a very different burden on those who are charged with responding to the query – the question in need of an answer. Whether sited in national call centres for mail-order goods or local units of *NHS Direct*, the isolated telephonist struggles to maintain her (for most are female) equilibrium within the pressurised environment of the answering 'service'. And the pressure to maintain the throughput – the number of calls answered per hour – is intense.

Robin Downie and Jane Macnaughton have asked what such a consumer-oriented ethic might do to those who are seeking to remain compassionate, beneficent and caring practitioners.[4] How does the world of teleworking undermine such a vocation, where consumers might seek to drive the agenda and demand a particular treatment, irrespective of the advice and wisdom of, for example, the doctor involved? And who ultimately will take responsibility for the transaction? In the market the seller must provide information on the goods, and perhaps advice, but the responsibility for buying the product, as well as for refusing to buy it, remains with the buyer. Is that how we see things happening in the world of healthcare?

The American film *Right to Reply* paints a picture of life lived through the medium of the telephone. The protagonists (apart from one couple at the end of the film) never meet face to face, but instead live their lives, even to the extent of being supported during childbirth, at the end of a mobile phone. Such networked existences challenge the old expectations of what it means to be family or community, of how to make sense of relating to others and to self, and of how to continue to be a humane doctor.

The service society

The historian and social commentator Theodore Zeldin believes that there are alternatives to such consumer-oriented societies. For him, the old-fashioned oriental bazaar, with its family-run businesses offering a mix of friendship and commercial activity, provides a valuable paradigm, where to share by drinking a cup of coffee with a prospective buyer is as important as making a sale.

> *The oriental bazaar is a reminder that humanity's evolution has not just been towards a consumer society, though abundance and prosperity for all is an almost universal goal. The other side of our evolution has been towards a service society, in which personal knowledge – almost intimacy with one's customers – is essential.*[5]

According to Zeldin's view of the world, economic institutions (of which a modern health service is but one example) must begin to take more account of the true needs and desires of all – not least those who are perceived to be in the ascendancy, namely the consumers. His *service society* opens up one alternative perspective.

Such a model of a service society can seem instantly appealing, suggesting that in the activity of being served there is benefit to both servant and recipient. This ideal pictures the vendor as emotionally and economically connected to the recipient or customer. Indeed, Zeldin writes of personal knowledge of the customer as verging on '*intimacy*' and being a necessity. He contrasts this type of relationship with the consumer who '*can buy anonymously without a word to the cashier*'.

Elsewhere Zeldin has written about the aspirations of the modern generation, who look for a new way of finding personal satisfaction in the workplace:

> *Many more of the new generation are saying that getting a job is not enough for them; they want a job that is fulfilling, useful to others, and involves contact with interesting people.*[6]

This desire for meaning and social contact at work coincides with a time when middle-class professions have ceased to be as liberating as they once were. '*Their members complain that the pleasures of their work are ruined by stress and that they are not properly respected or understood.*'

Human beings need to feel valued. It may be difficult to maintain the respect and understanding of others consistently, yet earning one's self-respect is fundamental to achieving a balanced sense of self-worth. On the whole, young people do not enter medical school solely in order to gain prestige and receive the praise of others. Yet it is unclear to what extent the ancient virtues of altruism and vocation have really featured in medical school life.

Altruism and idealism

Altruism has long been held to be a necessary attribute of the healthcare professional. Prospective medical students know it is important (and often manifest it privately), but paradoxically are advised to avoid speaking about it, or listing it as an essential part of their aspirations, during a medical school interview:

> *To the typical interview question, 'Why do you want to become a doctor?', applicants are warned, 'Answers that will turn your interviewers' stomachs and may lead to instant*

*rejection are: "I want to heal the sick"; "I want to care for my fellow human beings"'.
Instead, 'Start by stressing the importance of aspects that can be taught and, in particular,
emphasise the technical qualities that a doctor needs: the ability to carry out a thorough
medical examination, to diagnose accurately and quickly what is wrong, and the skill to
organise the correct treatment'.*[7]

This is an odd state of affairs. How can it be that talk of personal motivation to help and
to heal is so frowned upon? What is it that happens during medical training to shift
perceptions and perspectives so dramatically? The anthropologist and psychiatrist Simon
Sinclair experienced this same shift in sensibility when he revisited his medical training,
this time wearing his anthropological hat. Sitting in the audience among those considering a medical career, he noted that during a question-and-answer session about
forthcoming interviews, the clear message from the assembled panel of medical students
was that *'personal idealism is not something to show'.*[8]

Sinclair developed his disposition of 'idealism' from Howard Becker's work on
interviewing American medical students,[9] where prospective doctors speak of their
initial desires as follows: *'we want to help people ... upholding medical ideals'.* However, as the
years pass, this early idealism is replaced by later disillusionment, even within their time
as medical students, when gaining 'status' within the medical hierarchy takes on greater
importance, at least for the men. After all, *'medicine is the best of the professions'*, and
finding the best and most prestigious career within medicine itself must offer the greatest
rewards. There is therefore a tension between the high ideal of altruistic service on the
one hand, and the compelling call to achieve status within the medical profession, and
in society in general, on the other.

Altruism, service and vocation

What about the idea of altruism itself? The psychotherapist Robert Hale points out that,
on occasion, altruism can act as a defence mechanism, protecting doctors from conflict
and anxiety as well as providing an outlet for self-giving to others. Moreover, altruism
may be dangerous, as doctors feel an overwhelming call to be there and to care for their
patients, whatever the cost to themselves or others.[10]

However, Carl Whitehouse expresses a different viewpoint:

> *It seemed sad that a professional vocation should be seen as a key and altruism as no more
> than a defence which gave way under stress. This may be true for post-modern people, but
> what about the Good Samaritan?*[11]

Whitehouse asks whether there is still a place for the type of radical charity that was
exemplified by the Good Samaritan of Jesus' teaching, who went out of his way to provide
for a fellow traveller who had been brutally attacked and robbed.

Yet the Samaritan of the parable did not himself stay to watch over the recovery of the
invalid. Instead he moved on, leaving money so that others might care for the victim's

needs. Perhaps this is a picture of how to balance both personal engagement and delegation to others in our own quests to respond to the needs of others.

The notion of vocation suggests a calling to a role, or way of life, in which individuals become aware of the traditions that have shaped their chosen profession. For general practitioners, that means '*seeing themselves as part of the bigger picture, as those set apart, with others, to serve the community*'.[10] Those with a vocation can, of course, be abused – both by their employers and by the communities which they are called to serve. Service *per se* will ultimately be overwhelmed in the absence of a proper balance in the relationship between servant and served. This mutuality can be expressed in the language of covenant.

The covenant society

The risk of a service society is that the servant will become crushed by all that needs to be done. Today's general practitioners within the NHS feel the pressure of an unending supply of patients and paperwork and, more recently, of committees and meetings. Where will it all end? And is it still possible to talk of general practice as a vocation, of vocational training for GPs?

> *Talk of vocation seems to conjure up an image of the individual pitted against the potentially limitless task of serving humanity. Vocation, in this sense, is experienced as a heavy load. Vocation needs, rather, to be conceived as a three-dimensional relationship between persons.*[12]

The three persons (or parties) envisaged in such a covenant are mutually interdependent. The first party is the *caller*, who identifies a need in society and sets out to find (call) someone to meet that need. Such a party might be an institution, a charitable organisation or a philanthropist. The caller seeks out someone who is able to respond to the identified need. Such a person might be a doctor, teacher or priest. This second party is termed the *called*. The third party is the person (or persons) whose need is met by the actions of those who are called to their aid. They are termed *those to whom the called is sent* (*see* Box 2.3). Most importantly in this relationship, the arrangement between the three parties is established not through the bureaucratic and impersonal terms of a contract, but through the more personal and supple terms of what is termed a covenant.[13]

Box 2.3:   The three parties to a covenant

- The *caller* – identifies a need and commissions someone else to respond in action.
- The *called* – hears the 'call' and sets out to meet the identified need.
- *Those to whom the called is sent* – possess the unmet need and wait for help.

On hearing the summons (the call), the individual responds with a promise to obey. The terms of this promise literally constitute the individual as a 'professional' – one who professes, in this case a willingness to do the work ahead. This subsequent work is authorised and governed by the terms of the covenant – the terms of his or her profession.

In the medical context, the person who is called faces the distress of the ill and needy on a daily basis. This is a daunting prospect and can overwhelm the doctor unless there is a balancing voice – someone who can call a halt to overwork and overcommitment. In a covenant relationship, that is the role of the caller, who will arbitrate and see fair play, and who is obliged to ensure that the one who is called (in this case the vocational doctor) will not be destroyed by the magnitude of the task. This avoids a one-dimensional dynamic in which an unequal yoke is placed on the doctor, at the mercy of an ocean of patient need, where the doctor's response would be either to seek to withdraw by setting limits (perhaps via a contract), or to collapse under the strain. Equally, the caller ensures that the patients receive acceptable levels of care and treatment (*see* Figure 2.1).

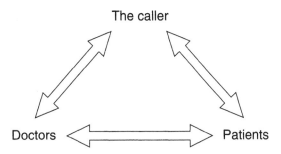

Figure 2.1 Parties to a covenant in healthcare.

Who then could act as the caller in a nationalised health service, to ensure reasonable and realistic goals and possibilities in the relationship between the called (the doctors) and the community to whom the doctors are sent (the patients). Direct employers and governments struggle to act as even-handed callers, driven as they are by the demands of electorates on the one hand and performance targets (and possibly shareholders) on the other. It is a better option to seek out an individual, organisation or independent body that is able to stand apart from this complex agenda and arbitrate with integrity as the representative of society at large.

Such an arbitrator would need to be aware of historical expressions of the doctor's ethical stance (e.g. the Hippocratic Oath), mainstream ethical viewpoints (e.g. those of the great religions and philosophies) and the perceptions of people of goodwill. A body with such views could then inform the debate, establishing and disseminating what would be the reasonable and acceptable expectations and responsibilities of both doctors and patients. This new body would need to be separate from the General Medical Council (which currently regulates doctors), the National Institute for Clinical Excellence (which sets standards of care) and the Commission for Health Improvement (which monitors whether those standards are achieved). Its task would be to monitor the new 'bargain' between the doctor and the patient, in order to ensure that those who are called and those to whom they are called continue to trust one another's motives and understand each other's point of view.

It would not be unreasonable to propose that the newly emerging primary care groups (PCGs) and primary care trusts (PCTs) consider this role (of caller) for themselves. Uniquely, they embrace doctors, patients, managers, others in primary healthcare, and representatives from Social Services. The PCTs in England have boards constituted with doctors in the minority. Their responsibility is to commission services and integrate care for all in the community. They are well placed to understand the pressures on practitioners and the needs of patients. It would appear that no one else is in that position. As long as vested interests are put to one side, and political interference (and politicisation) is nullified, PCGs and PCTs could act as callers in effective covenant relationships throughout primary care.

Conclusion

Traditionally, family doctors have been there for others, offering personal support and advice to patients and their families. In this role they manifest an ancient expression of the physician as one who touches, heals and cares. Where no cure is possible, they remain as a wise and trusted friend – the *amicus mortis – one who tells you the bitter truth and stays with you to the inexorable end.*[14]

GPs today are challenged to meet the needs of the whole of society – a society where consumerism, expectations of personal service and the speed of communication are all so dominant. At the same time, GPs must find new ways of maintaining their own identity, values and ethos in a world which struggles with the traditional professional ideals of vocation, altruism and covenant. Responding to such an agenda is not an easy task.

Summary points

- Consumerism is a dominant contemporary force.
- Managing demand for health and healthcare is difficult when expectations are high.
- Modern communication challenges historic ways of working.
- Providing service is rewarding, but there is a risk that it will drain practitioners.
- The 'bargain' between patients and doctors needs to be renegotiated.
- Mutually beneficial covenant relationships point one way ahead.

References

1   Harrison J and Innes R (2000) The end of certainty: professionalism re-visited. In: T van Zwanenberg and J Harrison (eds) *Clinical Governance in Primary Care.* Radcliffe Medical Press, Oxford.

2   Miles S (1998) *Consumerism – As a Way of Life.* Sage, London.

3   Gabriel Y and Lang T (1995) *The Unmanageable Consumer: Contemporary Consumption and its Fragmentations.* Sage, London.

4   Downie RS and Macnaughton J (2000) *Clinical Judgement. Evidence in Practice.* Oxford University Press, Oxford.

5   Zeldin T (1998) *Conversation.* The Harvill Press, London.

6   Zeldin T (1999) How work can be made less frustrating and conversation less boring. *BMJ.* **319**: 1633–5.

7   Ruston J (1993) *Getting into Medical School.* Trotman, Richmond.

8   Sinclair S (1997) *Making Doctors. An Institutional Apprenticeship.* Berg, Oxford.

9   Becker HS, Geer B, Hughes EC *et al.* (1961) *Boys In White: Student Culture in Medical School.* University of Chicago Press, Chicago.

10   Harrison J (1998) Regaining control. In: J Harrison and T van Zwanenberg (eds) *GP Tomorrow.* Radcliffe Medical Press, Oxford.

11   Whitehouse C (1999) Review of GP Tomorrow. *Triple Helix.* **7**: 22.

12   Harrison J and Innes R (1997) *Medical Vocation and Generation X.* Grove Books, Cambridge.

13   May WF (1983) *The Physician's Covenant: Images of the Healer in Medical Ethics.* Westminster Press, Philadelphia, PA.

14   Illich I (1995) Death undefeated. *BMJ.* **311**: 1652–3.

CHAPTER THREE

Professional regulation

Tim van Zwanenberg and Cath O'Halloran

Professional men, they have no cares;
Whatever happens, they get theirs.

Ogden Nash

> This chapter describes the origins and nature of a profession, and explores ideas about professional knowledge and expertise. New professions emerged in the twentieth century, and the status of professions and their relationship with the State has changed. A new agreement between medicine and society about the regulation of the medical profession is in the process of being negotiated.

The rationale for professions

George Bernard Shaw (with his famous quote that *All professions are conspiracies against the laity*) is not the only person to have been cynical about the self-interest of professional groups. Yet another great social observer from the nineteenth century, Charles Dickens, did much to bring the issues which govern the rationale for professions to public attention. For example, in his preface to *The First Cheap Edition of Nicholas Nickleby*, 1848, he set out some of his views on professions with particular respect to teachers.[1] The book incidentally had a profound effect on the schools parodied by his description of the 'internal economy of Dotheboys Hall' and its proprietor Mr Wackford Squeers.

> *Although any man who had proved his unfitness for any other occupation in life was free, without examination or qualification, to open a school anywhere, although preparation for the functions he*

undertook was required in the surgeon who assisted to bring a boy into the world, or might one day assist, perhaps, to send him out of it, – in the chemist, the attorney, the butcher, the baker, the candle-stick maker, – the whole round of crafts and trades, the schoolmaster excepted, and although schoolmasters, as a race, were the blockheads and impostors that might naturally be expected to arise from such a state of things, and to flourish in it, these Yorkshire schoolmasters were the lowest and most rotten round in the whole ladder. Traders in the avarice, indifference or imbecility of parents, and the helplessness of children; ignorant, sordid, brutal men, to whom few considerate persons would have entrusted the board and lodging of a horse or a dog, they formed the worthy corner-stone of a structure which, for absurdity and a magnificent high-handed laissez-aller neglect, has rarely been exceeded in the world.

We hear sometimes of an action for damages against the unqualified medical practitioner, who has deformed a broken limb in pretending to heal it. But what about the hundreds of thousands of minds that have been deformed for ever by the incapable pettifoggers who have pretended to form them!

Among other things, this passage illustrates that many of the controversial issues relating to education have persisted to the present day – for example, parental choice and the effect of the market, teachers' professionalism and competence, school effectiveness, and the treatment of children in care. Of more relevance, 140 years on from Dickens' time and the inception of professional self-regulation for doctors, a General Teaching Council (GTC) for England has only just been established. In comparison, the Medical (Registration) Act of 1858 established the General Medical Council (GMC) to regulate the profession of medicine (to which Dickens also alludes), and to maintain a register of all medical practitioners.

Prior to that there had been three types of medical attendant, each with their own form of regulation. These were the physicians, who were members of a 'learned profession', the surgeons, who were skilled craftsmen, and the apothecaries, who were tradesmen who dispensed medicines. With the industrial revolution and rapid advances in science, the traditional boundaries became blurred (reminiscent of the blurring of roles among health professionals today). General practitioners owe their origins to all three groups, and were first called surgeon apothecaries. Indeed, membership of the Royal College of Surgeons was a standard qualification for GPs who, even today, practise from surgeries. The Medical (Registration) Act had been preceded by the Apothecaries Act of 1815.

Although the passage from *Nicholas Nickleby* is expressed in Dickens' typical prose, he does identify a number of the principles which have underpinned the concept of profession, namely fitness for occupation, examination, qualification, trust, and protection from charlatans for the innocent and vulnerable. He was also clearly of the view that regulation could not be left to market forces, or to 'high-handed *laissez-aller* neglect' as he put it! Yet until the 1950s there were traditionally only two professions, namely medicine and the law (if one discounts prostitution, which is said to be the 'oldest profession'), and the role of the State in the regulation of these two professions was negligible. Was it that medicine and law were perceived to have power over life and death, and were thus accorded special status because of their mystique?

The nature of a profession

The profession of medicine has been in existence for hundreds of years, stretching back long before Dickens' time, and present-day general practitioners rarely stop to think about the implications of being a member of a profession as they go about their busy professional lives. However, events at the turn of the millennium have raised questions about the regulation of the profession of medicine, and how doctors are held to account for their practice.[2] The Law Society (the body which self-regulates the profession of law) has similarly been criticised by the Lord Chancellor for its vast backlog of unresolved complaints against lawyers.

Against this background it is worth pausing to reconsider what it is that characterises a profession. How, for example, in these utilitarian days does a profession differ from a job? How is it that other groups (e.g. teachers and nurses) have only become professions in the last 50 years?

An historical description of the nature of a profession from the sixteenth century identifies seven characteristics[3] (*see* Box 3.1). However, the concept of profession is not static, but instead represents a dynamic relationship between the group of experts, their clients and the State. Thus although the characteristics from medieval times are still recognisable today, the nature of each characteristic has changed over time with the changing interests and relative power of the three parties.

Box 3.1:   The characteristics of a profession (circa sixteenth century)

1   There should be a relationship of trust and confidence with the client.
2   An element of public service and duty to the community should be present.
3   It should relate to an area of well-defined knowledge, to include theoretical knowledge.
4   A period of training is usually provided, often in an institution.
5   It is organised and institutionalised both to test the competence of members and to maintain it.
6   It is a social group with its own hierarchy, social life and commitment.
7   It claims and is accorded status based on salary, learning acquired at the highest grade, organisation and solidarity, code of conduct and professional ethics, and independence.

In the 1950s there was considerable debate about the attributes and traits of a profession, perhaps because of the desire of other groups to extend profession beyond medicine and the law. Box 3.2 lists the features of a profession from that time. A number of points are worth noting. First, there is really no mention of the consumers. Secondly, clients' needs are defined by the practitioner. Thirdly, there is an underlying principle of 'let the buyer trust', rather than 'let the buyer beware'. Finally, most doctors, through their engagement with the NHS, had by then foregone their right to charge a fee, except from their private patients.

Box 3.2:   The attributes of a profession (circa 1950)

These include the following:
1   monopoly over practice
2   the existence of an organised body responsible for:
    • entry and training
    • licence to practise
    • ethical code of conduct
    • standards of practice
3   independence of judgement and practice
4   practitioners practise individually – linked loosely with colleagues
5   the professional–client relationship is central
6   disinterested services to the public (i.e. altruistic)
7   long period of training, with high academic prowess
8   discrete body of expert knowledge (both theoretical and applied)
9   expert skill base
10   a negotiable fee is charged
11   high social status and income.

New professions and changing status

As the new professions (sometimes called semi-professions by sociological commentators) started to emerge in the 1960s, it became clear that they did not fit neatly into the framework of professional attributes which described medicine and the law. There were questions about whether the new professions were truly based on an expert body of knowledge. Their training was much shorter, and the academic requirements of their members were much less. They were not so obviously an elite social group, and they were subject to much greater levels of government control. Thus professions started to be seen in functional terms (i.e. they provided an expert service, which recipients were not expert enough to evaluate). However, it was also clear that members of these new professions gained in social and probably also economic standing.

Since the 1970s, the professions have come to be viewed as political phenomena, and their political power has been attacked from a variety of angles. Some have seen the professions as threatening individual citizens' ability to assume responsibility for themselves, alleging that the professions' determination of clients' needs is merely a device to sustain their own power. An example of this might be the groups who have lobbied the obstetric establishment to promote natural childbirth. Others have been concerned that the professions have undue influence on national political structures, and view professions as part of the 'democratic deficit'. Yet others have argued that professional codes of conduct have done little to provide clients with redress for their dissatisfaction, and that self-regulation merely protects the interests of the members.

Thus professionalism has come to be viewed as an ideology – a political stratagem for securing a niche in the market and for gaining power and status.

By the 1980s, the professions were under attack both from the political left (who believed that the welfare state was assisting the middle classes to become a self-perpetuating elite), and from the political right (who wanted to open up restrictive practices to market forces). Thus it was that the 'New Right' Thatcher government of the 1980s and 1990s set about changing the relationship between the State and the professions. This was particularly evident in education, where a raft of legislation has fundamentally altered the working lives of teachers. This radical programme of change with respect to professional groups, particularly those in the public sector, seems set to continue under the 'New Labour' government.

So far as medicine is concerned, clear changes can be seen in the interests of the three parties – the profession, the patients and the State – and in the dominant themes of the time (*see* Table 3.1).

Table 3.1 The changing interests

Dominant theme	State	Patients	Profession
Exploitation of the vulnerable	No interest	Exploitation of the ignorant and vulnerable	Seeking professional identity (against charlatans)
Protection of the vulnerable	Protection of the vulnerable Medical Act 1848	Increasing education Universal suffrage	Expert knowledge Specialised service
Provision of services	National Insurance Act 1911 Inception of NHS 1948	Entitlement (limited) Universally free at the point of delivery	Code of practice, ethics, integrity Self-regulation (conduct only)
Profession as self-serving elite	Value for money Variation in quality Inequalities in health	Informed consumers Explicit rights Higher incomes Expert patients	Post-NHS rights to private practice Protection of members' power and status
Democratic deficit	Confronting powerful groups (e.g. unions and professions) Failures of self-regulation Control by legislation, protocol and inspection (e.g. Office for Standards in Education (OFSTED) NICE and CHI)	Involvement in 'patient partnership' Access to expert knowledge (e.g. the Internet) Self-help and patient representative groups	Publication of *Good Medical Practice* GMC Health Committee GMC Performance Committee
Adjustment	Media 'spin'	Media influence	Revalidation GMC changes

Medical professionalism

Schon, in his review of professional education, refers to the observation made by Everett Hughes, a sociologist of the professions, that the professions had struck a bargain with society.[4] In return for access to their extraordinary knowledge in matters of great human importance, society has granted them a mandate for social control in their fields of specialisation, a high degree of autonomy in their practice, and a licence to determine who shall assume the mantle of professional autonomy. Sir Donald Irvine, President of the GMC, has suggested that in the current climate of an apparent loss of confidence in the professions, the time has come to renegotiate this bargain.[5] He suggests that if the trust of patients in the competence of their doctors is not re-established and maintained, then state regulation will be the price paid by the profession. The Chief Medical Officer has also warned that self-regulation is a privilege.[6]

Medical professionalism is said to rest on expertise, ethics and service.[7] The continuation of independent self-regulation depends on the following criteria:

1   there is such an unusual degree of knowledge and skill involved in medical work that non-professionals are not equipped to evaluate or regulate it[8]
2   doctors can be trusted to work responsibly, and the profession can be trusted to act when members fail to perform competently or ethically.[7]

Professional knowledge

The possession of expert knowledge and skill has always been one of the defining characteristics of membership of a profession, but there has long been debate about the nature of this knowledge and its relationship to skilled practice. In medicine in particular, the development of a scientific knowledge base was clearly desirable. However, the relationship between the body of scientific medical knowledge and the skilled practice of a general practitioner in their surgery is extremely complex.

Medicine as science

The emergence of the natural sciences, scientific investigation and the study of the human body in the eighteenth and nineteenth centuries lead to medicine being viewed as a science. The visible culmination of this movement is the Human Genome Project. As the structure and functions of the human body and the mechanisms of disease were discovered, so the role of scientific knowledge in underpinning practice was established. Medical schools became associated with universities and adopted their academic values. Students studied medical science first and then, during a subsequent period of supervised clinical practice, they would learn to apply research-based techniques to diagnosis, treatment and prevention. Physicians were thus trained as scientific problem-solvers.

In this hierarchy of knowledge, basic science is placed above applied science, which in turn is placed above the skills of day-to-day practice. Broadly speaking, the greater one's proximity to basic science, the higher one's academic status. This may explain general practice's past struggle to be accepted as an academic discipline.

Medicine as practice

Aristotle had drawn a distinction between 'technical knowledge', which was capable of being written down, and 'practical knowledge', which was expressed only in practice. More recently, Eraut has taken this classification further, proposing two forms of professional knowledge, namely codified knowledge (knowing what) and personal knowledge (knowing how).[9] Codified knowledge is published in scientific journals, textbooks, 'how to do it' manuals, university curricula and examination syllabuses.

Personal knowledge consists of codified knowledge that has been transformed into a personalised form through use in practice, the procedural knowledge that supports skilled behaviour, the deliberative processes associated with clinical reasoning, and the experiential knowledge that the practitioner builds up from noticing recurring events (pattern recognition). Personal knowledge is highly individualised and not easily articulated. The professional is unaware of much of what they know.

Practice as professional artistry

The proposition that medical practice is founded on 'personal' knowledge does not fit well with the scientific problem-solving model, but may reflect reality.

> In the varied topography of professional practice, there is a high, hard ground overlooking a swamp. On the high ground, manageable problems lend themselves to solution through the application of research-based theory and technique. In the swampy lowland, messy, confusing problems defy technical solution. The irony of this situation is that the problems of the high ground tend to be relatively unimportant to individuals or society at large, however great their technical interest may be, while in the swamp lie the problems of greatest human concern. The practitioner must choose. Shall he remain on the high ground where he can solve relatively unimportant problems according to prevailing standards of rigor, or shall he descend to the swamp of important problems and non-rigorous inquiry?[4]

Schon has developed this alternative view of professional practice even further, coining the term 'professional artistry'. He describes artistry as an exercise of intelligence – a kind of knowing. In professional practice, applied science and research-based technique occupy a critically important but limited territory, bounded on all sides by artistry. This artistry is concerned with framing problems and implementing solutions. Improvisation is needed to mediate the use of applied science in practice (see Box 3.3). Schon's notion of artistry echoes Aristotle's 'practical knowledge', but he claims that the knowledge in professional artistry is not inherently mysterious, but that it can be learned by the careful study of the performance of skilled practitioners.[4]

Box 3.3: An example of 'professional artistry' from general practice

A normally fit young man consults his GP with a three-day history of pain in his left hand. On examination, the GP finds the classic signs of Dupuytren's contracture, which she estimates must have been present for months. The diagnosis is easy and no active treatment is required, at least for the foreseeable future. It appears to be a straightforward case where the GP simply needs to inform the patient of the diagnosis, treatment and prognosis and send him quickly on his way.

However, the experienced GP will consider a number of factors beyond the simple diagnosis of a minor condition. These might include the following examples.

- Dupuytren's contracture does not normally cause pain. Is the patient only able to present to his doctor with pain rather than 'deformity'?
- The signs suggest that the condition has been present and worsening for months. Has the patient been denying it to himself?
- If so, what has provoked him to attend now?
- How has his eventual acknowledgement that something is wrong affected his image of himself as a fit and well man?
- What does he fear – being 'deformed', being 'ill', being in need of treatment?
- Is he worried that the condition will spread to other parts of his body, or that it is infectious?
- Or is he worried that his delay in seeking advice may mean that it is too late for effective treatment?
- The doctor needs to explore these questions very sensitively.
- The doctor needs to 'break the bad news' that there is something wrong, and do this in a way which allows the patient to accept it.
- Finally, the doctor needs to 'check out' that the patient understands, and to offer support in the future.

At first glance this appears to be a simple case. In fact, it requires a high level of professional skill.

Medical decision making

The way in which doctors make decisions has interested researchers from several fields. The early studies concentrated on identifying the features that distinguished between good and poor diagnosticians. The main findings were that experts know no more codified knowledge than do novices. Indeed, recall of biomedical knowledge peaks at the time of initial qualification and tails off with experience. In contrast, skilled performance depends on knowledge that is organised into clinically useful forms.

More recently, decision theory has been explored. This involves constructing mathematical models to determine the relative merits of different decisions.[10] These models deal with probabilities. An example might be a doctor considering whether to prescribe a drug (known to cause severe side-effects in a proportion of patients) to a patient suffering from a condition which has multiple risk factors. Out of this work has emerged the approach that we now call evidence-based medicine (EBM). The double-blind randomised control trial (RCT) has become the gold standard for research design, because meta-analyses of such studies are the best way of generating the data which support decision theory modelling and thus EBM. However, meta-analyses only calculate the odds more accurately.

Professional knowledge in general practice

How much of a GP's practice can be modelled in this way? We are back in the swamp. Skilled general practice depends on a (still poorly understood) combination of learned rules and sufficient clinical experience, and not even the EBM evangelists suggest that all areas of general practice could be covered by guidelines derived from RCTs. Individual GPs interpret the rules in the light of their own clinical experience, but inevitably this interpretation is a potential source of error in the individual case.

As the codified knowledge of medicine has advanced, so paradoxically the traditional view of the GP has changed. He or she is no longer the expert, who has knowledge that is not available to or understood by the patient. The codified knowledge of medicine is now readily available to patients. However, in practice rapid decisions still have to be made about extremely complex phenomena in a climate of uncertainty. Scientific advances may reduce uncertainty in some areas of practice, or support guidelines which help to unravel complexity in others. However, in many areas of practice the doctor will legitimately select a course of action from their repertoire that has produced a good outcome in similar circumstances in the past.

Professional regulation

Replacing one area of professional mystique (codified knowledge about the workings of the human body) with another (professional artistry) will not meet the demands of the public and the State in the present climate. This is well recognised by most doctors, although many have been frustrated by the apparent ineffectiveness of the GMC on the one hand and by adverse political and media comment on the other. Each high-profile case of professional misconduct or incompetence has brought forth calls for the end of self-regulation, yet the GMC has done much to bolster its role over the last few years.

The General Medical Council

Until the 1980s, the GMC simply registered all doctors on qualification, and concerned itself with breaches of their professional conduct (i.e. adultery with patients, advertising, and so on). Even now, patients and doctors find it difficult to believe that for the first 100 or so years of its existence the Council barely addressed doctors' competence. The first development of note was the introduction of the health procedures – an acknowledgement that illness could subvert professional practice.

During the 1990s a series of developments followed. Working closely with the universities and the Medical Royal Colleges, the GMC began to develop and introduce 'explicit standards of professional practice' (*Duties of a Doctor: Good Medical Practice*),[11] a new curriculum in the medical schools (*Tomorrow's Doctors: Recommendations on Undergraduate Medical Education*)[12] and changes to the pre-registration year (*The New Doctor: Recommendations on General Clinical Training*).[13] Performance was added to conduct and health, with the introduction of the performance procedures through the Medical (Professional Performance) Act 1995. To support this, the GMC developed a means of assessing clinical performance in poorly performing doctors at their place of work. Those who were found to exhibit an unacceptable pattern of performance could be arraigned before the GMC and either struck off the register or compelled to undergo remedial training. Furthermore, legislation was enacted to prolong the period of suspension from the register before a struck-off doctor could apply for reinstatement. A major overhaul of the GMC's structure, constitution and governance was also promised.[14]

Revalidation

Finally in the summer of the year 2000 the GMC set forth its proposals for the revalidation of all doctors.[15] This represented a radical departure from all that had gone before – a watershed in the history of the regulation of the medical profession. Prior to this the GMC, in fulfilling its duty to Parliament to make sure that those admitted to the Medical Register were competent, relied on the combination of an historical record of a doctor's initial qualification and responses to complaints about practice. The system assumed that doctors would keep their practice up to date throughout their professional lives. With revalidation, doctors will now have to demonstrate on a periodic and regular basis that they remain fit to practise in their chosen field.

Revalidation for GPs will be based on the criteria and minimum standards set out in *Good Medical Practice for General Practitioners* – the version of the GMC's *Good Medical Practice* that is customised for clinical general practice (*see* Chapter 8). Meanwhile, GPs who aspire to higher than minimum standards will have a menu of accredited awards from the Royal College of General Practitioners (RCGP) to aim for. These include Membership (MRCGP) by examination or assessment, Fellowship (FRCGP) by assessment, accredited professional development (APD) and the Quality Practice Award (QPA).

Quality assurance in the NHS

The professional regulation of doctors (and nurses and other professional groups) is only one element of quality assurance in the NHS. Individual clinicians work as members of both clinical teams and of larger organisations. Healthcare for individual patients is increasingly based on teamworking. Under these circumstances, organisations and teams need mechanisms to ensure quality beyond the individual practitioner. Mistakes and tragedies occur as often due to system failure as they ever do through individual poor performance.

Clinical governance is being introduced to support this collective (as opposed to individual) quality assurance, and offers a coherent framework for bringing together the various disparate quality improvement activities (e.g. clinical audit, continuing professional development, learning from complaints) (*see* Chapter 9). Professional regulation then needs to be viewed as part of a continuum, starting with the individual doctor and extending through the clinical team to the healthcare organisation (i.e. practice or primary care trust).

Quality in the public services

The present government has made much of its efforts to demonstrate 'joined-up thinking'. By this it means that its policies are consistent with one another. From this point of view it is interesting to compare the approaches to professional regulation and quality assurance across the two main public services, namely health and education. Table 3.2 shows such a comparison using the framework from *A First-Class Service: Quality in the New NHS.*[16]

Table 3.2 Quality enhancement in public services

Quality mechanism	National Health Service	Education services
Clear standards of service	National Institute of Clinical Excellence National Service Frameworks	Standards and Effectiveness Unit National Curriculum School Curriculum and Assessment Authority
Dependable local delivery	Professional self-regulation Clinical governance Lifelong learning	General Teaching Council Teacher Training Agency National numeracy and literacy hours Standards Task Force In-Service Training (INSET)
Monitored standards	Commission for Health Improvement National Performance Framework National Patient and User Survey	Office for Standards in Education (OFSTED)

It is not possible to map each agency or process exactly across the two services, but the similarities are apparent. For example, both the national curriculum and national service frameworks outline what should be done. However, for teachers the imposition of literacy and numeracy hours goes much further – they are being told not only what to teach, but also how to teach it. On the other hand, the very recent establishment of a General Teaching Council, which will register teachers in England (Scotland has had its own GTC since 1965), contrasts markedly with the plans to enhance professional self-regulation in the NHS.

The Commission for Health Improvement will be visiting NHS organisations over a three- to four-yearly cycle to inspect their arrangements for clinical governance. This is not dissimilar to the role of the Office for Standards in Education (OFSTED), although it involves entering the fray at a much later point in contemporary history and with (as yet) a much lower profile. It remains to be seen whether the commission will assume as important a role as OFSTED has in education.

Conclusion

The President of the GMC has described the emergence of a new and explicit culture of professionalism in medicine. Medicine is inherently a judgement-based profession, but by putting patient safety first this new culture would minimise the risks of clinical error. The President of the GMC believes that it will achieve this by 'replacing blame, secrecy and misplaced professional solidarity with the attitudes, language and habits of quality improvement'. Openness is said to be the key.[14]

In the longer term it remains to be seen whether doctors can regulate themselves effectively to the satisfaction of their patients and the government. The nature of professional regulation in medicine appears to have changed from an intra-medical concern (the measurement of standards by peers, the control of competition, and so on) to primarily justifying professional competence to the public (as part of the bargain of professional privilege). We are thus moving from doctor–doctor regulation to patient–doctor regulation, from paternalistic beneficence to citizenship, and from patient dependence to qualified autonomy.

One of the most important philosophical problems underlying professional regulation is the clash between profession-based ethics and the ever-growing legal rights to self-determination. Being a patient might necessarily entail some sacrifice of personal rights to self-determination 'for one's own good'.

Summary points

- Until the 1950s there were only two professions, namely medicine and the law, and the role of the State in their regulation was negligible.
- The concept of a profession has changed over time, with new professions such as teaching and nursing emerging.
- The status of a profession represents an agreement between the group of experts and their clients and the State. In return for autonomy and control over their affairs, the profession maintains standards and protects the vulnerable from exploitation.
- The possession of expert knowledge and skill is one of the defining characteristics of profession, but there is debate about the nature of this knowledge and its relationship to skilled practice.
- Recent high-profile cases of misconduct and incompetence have brought medical self-regulation into question.
- In recent years the GMC has developed a range of initiatives, culminating in its proposals for revalidation.
- The government has also introduced new quality assurance structures and processes in the NHS, and similarly in education.

References

1 Dickens C (1848, recent paperback edition 1985) *Nicholas Nickleby*. Penguin, Harmondsworth.

2 Pringle M (2000) The Shipman inquiry: implications for the public's trust in doctors. *Br J Gen Pract*. **50**: 355–6.

3 Lello J (1993) *Accountability in Practice*. Cassell, London.

4 Schon DA (1987) *Educating the Reflective Practitioner: Toward a New Design for Teaching and Learning in the Professions*. Jossey-Bass Inc., San Francisco, CA.

5 Irvine D (1999) The performance of doctors: the new professionalism. *Lancet*. **353**: 1174–7.

6 Department of Health (1999) *Supporting Doctors, Protecting Patients. A Consultation Paper on Preventing, Recognising and Dealing With Poor Clinical Performance of Doctors in England*. Department of Health, London.

7 Irvine D (1997) The performance of doctors. I. Professionalism and self-regulation in a changing world. *BMJ*. **314**: 1540–2.

8 Friedson E (1988) *Profession of Medicine: a Study of the Sociology of Applied Knowledge*. University of Chicago Press, London.

9 Eraut M (1994) *Developing Professional Knowledge and Competence*. Falmer Press, London.

10 Eraut M (2000) Non-formal learning and tacit knowledge in professional work. *Br J Educ Psychol*. **70**: 113–36.

11 General Medical Council (1995) *Duties of a Doctor: Good Medical Practice.* General Medical Council, London.

12 General Medical Council (1993) *Tomorrow's Doctors: Recommendations on Undergraduate Medical Education.* General Medical Council, London.

13 General Medical Council (1997) *The New Doctor: Recommendations on General Clinical Training.* General Medical Council, London.

14 General Medical Council (2000) *Changing Times. Changing Culture.* General Medical Council, London.

15 General Medical Council (2000) *Revalidating Doctors. Ensuring Standards, Securing the Future.* General Medical Council, London.

16 Department of Health (1998) *A First-Class Service: Quality in the New NHS.* Department of Health, London.

CHAPTER FOUR

Modernisation and New Labour

Rob Innes

We want to see healthier people in a healthier country. People improving their own health supported by communities working through local organisations against a backdrop of action by the government.

Secretary of State for Health, July 1999[1]

This chapter puts the challenges facing GPs in a political context. It shows how the values that inform New Labour's programme of modernisation compare with the traditional values of general practice. It unpacks what government means by 'modern' policies, structures and culture in the NHS, and it suggests ways in which the professional identity of the GP may need to change in order to respond to the contemporary political agenda.

The politics of the 'Third Way'

'*The government has a mission to modernise ... Modernisation is a hallmark of the Government.*'[2] New Labour has indeed put 'modernisation' at the heart of its political programme. It is a programme that covers our schools, hospitals, economy, criminal justice system, democratic framework and the structures of government themselves.[2,3] The intention is to produce institutions which are appropriate for the new conditions of a new millennium.

Some examples of these major conditions include the following:[4]

- a shift from manufacturing production to information technology[5]
- the death of socialism as a viable political option[6]

- the expansion of choice in consumption and lifestyle[7]
- the changing role of women[8]
- the dominance of global markets.[9]

The 'Third Way' has arisen as a response to these conditions. It is not unique to the UK, but has been adopted by politicians in the USA, Germany, France and Italy. In February 1998, Tony Blair spoke in Washington of his ambition to create an international consensus of the centre-left for the twenty-first century. He called for a new policy framework for a new global order. Third Way gurus argue that the new social conditions require nothing less than a complete rethinking of our social institutions.[10]

Certainly the Third Way has its critics. Those on the right regard it as vague and lacking content. '*All that is solid melts into Blair.*'[11] Those on the left see it as watered-down free-marketeering – Mrs Thatcher without the handbag. Yet at least in this country, the politics of the Third Way appear to be without serious challengers for the foreseeable future. Moreover, for all the complaints about lack of content, Blair's government is rolling out policies across a wide range of areas of national life, not least in the NHS, with far-reaching consequences. Like it or not, the modernising agenda of the Third Way affects us all and will probably be with us for some time to come.

For its advocates, the Third Way is an attempt to transcend both old-style socialism and the neoliberalism of recent Conservative governments. The politics of an earlier era polarised around economic questions – markets versus state ownership, the freedom of the individual versus obligations to the community, and opposing views on the role of the welfare state. The Third Way attempts to move beyond these binary oppositions by setting politics within the conditions of the 'modern' context. Anthony Giddens, allegedly Blair's favourite intellectual, sets out the following core values for the Third Way[12] (*see* Box 4.1).

Box 4.1:   Core values of the Third Way

Equality
Protection of the vulnerable
Freedom as autonomy
No rights without responsibilities
Cosmopolitan pluralism
Philosophic conservatism

Some of the traditional left-wing concerns remain, such as a commitment to equality and to protection of the vulnerable. However, there is also an emphasis on balancing rights and responsibilities. Here the Third Way moves beyond left-wing communitarianism and right-wing individualism. There is recognition of our contemporary plurality of lifestyles and life choices, and importantly there is the pragmatic recognition that the market is here to stay – a 'philosophic conservatism'. New Labour is not attempting the wholesale undoing of previous Conservative (neoliberal) reforms (*see* Box 4.2 for definitions of key political terms).

Box 4.2:   Key political '-isms'

Communitarianism	A social and political view which stresses the importance of the community in giving individuals a sense of identity and worth, and in the transmission of moral values. It has arisen in part as a reaction to individualism[13]
Conservatism	A cautious, pragmatic attitude towards reform in social and political life[14]
Individualism	A social and political view which starts with individuals. Society is an aggregate of individuals, and social institutions exist to serve individuals. The individualist esteems freedom and autonomy, and is sceptical of social solidarity and authority[15]
Modernisation	Strictly a term borrowed from sociology, which describes the process whereby primitive societies evolve into modern, industrialised societies, becoming more differentiated and complex in their social structure. The term has been given new content by politicians of the Third Way[16]
Neoliberalism	The revival of classical liberal ideas such as the importance of the individual, the limited role of the State, and the value of the free market. Linked to the political ideas of the so-called 'New Right'[17]
Pluralism	The toleration or acceptance of a diversity of opinions and values[18]
Socialism	A political and economic theory which advocates that the community as a whole should own the means of production, capital, land and property.[19]

New Labour and the professional GP

The values of socialism could never be expected to be wholly sympathetic to the professional doctor. In so far as socialists saw themselves as inheritors of Marx, doctors and other professional groups were always liable to be regarded as forces of reaction – bourgeois class enemies. But neither is neoliberalism sympathetic to professional groups. In thorough-going free-marketeering, doctors take their place as just one more producer group. Again they are liable to be regarded as reactionary – this time for opposing the introduction of management and markets into their professional relationships.

Might professional groups expect more support from New Labour? On taking office, Blair's 'philosophic conservatism' was expressed in a continuation of the management revolution in the NHS that had been started by Mrs Thatcher. For all that New Labour mocked John Major's Patients' Charter, it readily adopted the familiar charter themes of quality, responsiveness, customer empowerment and better public service.[20] As he set out a vision for his government, Blair declared:

> *On health, Labour's objective is a rebuilt public health system that promotes good health and an NHS rebuilt as a people's service, free of market dogma, but also free of the old and new bureaucratic constraints, serving all the people, with doctors, nurses and administrators working as part of a unified system.*[21]

This would be a government that was not inherently hostile to professional groups, but would certainly demand change from them. Box 4.3 compares the values of New Labour with those of traditional professional groups.

Box 4.3: Comparison of values

New Labour values	*Professional values*
Openness	Confidentiality
Equality	Respect for an elite
Quality (as defined by government)	Quality (as defined by the profession)
Management	Professional judgement
Political leadership	Professional leadership
Democratic accountability	Self-regulation
Teamworking	Maintenance of professional roles
Maximising service levels	Retention of control over service delivery
Partnership	Professional autonomy
Customer empowerment	Professional expertise
Modernisation	Conservatism
General health improvement	Commitment to individual patients/clients

---

Modernising policies

'Modernisation' seems, on the face of it, a pretty vacuous notion. Almost anything or anyone could make a claim to be 'modern' in their own way! However, in its statements and official papers, the Blair government has attached some quite specific content to the idea. Box 4.4 shows, in the left-hand column, key policy guidelines across Whitehall departments set out in the White Paper *Modernising Government* (1999).[22] The right-hand column lists examples of how these map on to policies and initiatives implemented within the particular domain of the National Health Service.[22]

Box 4.4:   Modernising policies

Modernising Government *policy guidelines*[22]	*Examples with regard to NHS policies/initiatives*
Pragmatic, not bound by 'old dogmas'	Private finance initiatives for new hospital buildings Using market mechanisms to extend the power of GP commissioning
Inclusive, both in policy formation and in service delivery	Three-year health improvement programmes to address inequality Health action zones New ways of delivering primary care (e.g. as walk-in centres)
Integrated 'joined-up government', co-ordination across traditionally disparate areas	Cross-departmental co-operation on public health NHS organisation to have a statutory duty of partnership PCGs required to work closely with local Social Services departments
Committed to quality	National Service Frameworks NICE evidence-based medicine guidelines Clinical governance Commission for Health Improvement
Information age	*NHS Direct* and *NHS Direct On-Line* PCs on every GP's desk
Long term	Targets for reduction in the number of deaths from cancer, coronary heart disease, stroke, accidents and suicide by the year 2010

Whether or not you agree with it, and whether or not it can deliver what it promises, the Third Way supplies an ideology which is every bit as radical as the traditional left- and right-wing options. 'Modernisation', when it is fleshed out, is a powerful ideology for change of quite a comprehensive kind.

Modern structures

GP fundholding ended with the Health Act receiving Royal Assent in July 1999. In place of the allegedly unfair NHS internal market, the government introduced primary care groups (PCGs) as the major unit responsible for delivering primary care to a locality.

PCGs are expected to serve, typically, about 100 000 patients, so around 500 PCGs would be needed to cover the whole country.

The government has stated that PCGs have three main aims:[23]

- health improvement – to improve the health of and address health inequalities in their communities
- developing primary and community health – by improving the quality of care through supporting GPs and other health providers in the delivery and integration of services
- commissioning secondary care services – to advise the health authority on (or assume responsibility for) the commissioning of hospital services for their patients.

This envisages a rather profound change in the role of the GP. GPs are now required to address themselves not just to the medical problems of individual patients, but to the overall health of the local community. GPs can expect to have a role in health promotion, public health, and reducing inequalities in health. The PCG can be held accountable for its performance through targets agreed with a local health authority via its Health Improvement Programme.

The PCG is responsible for the integration of services across GPs and other health providers. PCGs already constitute themselves in a range of ways to enable this to occur. One survey of the organisational status of PCGs found the following:[24]

- health authority subcommittee (public)
- prospective NHS trust (with access to PFI)
- legal partnership (independent)
- (not for profit) limited company (private)
- joint venture (commercial)
- charitable foundation (voluntary)
- local patients' association (community).

The government hopes that PCGs, particularly as they become self-governing primary care trusts (PCTs), will bring together all of the 'stakeholders' in health provision, including GPs, nurses, midwives, paramedics, Social Services and patient representatives. Moreover, some PCGs are already moving in the direction of becoming 'community organisations', with clients as enrolled members sharing in decision making about service provision rather than merely being registered patients who receive clinically prescribed treatments.[24]

The commissioning powers of primary care organisations have been substantially increased under recent legislation. Compared to previous fundholding practices, PCGs are now large enough to have real purchasing power in placing contracts with NHS trusts, and they may commission both elective and core services. The advent of PCTs signifies a major swing in resource control from secondary to primary care organisations.

A modern culture: clinical governance

'*Clinical governance is a quality concept*,'[25] according to Chief Medical Officer Liam Donaldson.

In the post-war years of the NHS, and into the 1960s and 1970s, the role, status and prestige of the doctor were their own guarantees of quality. Formal methods of quality assurance did not appear in the NHS until after the Griffiths Recommendations for General Management (1983) – the 'first wave' of Conservative managerial reform.[26] The notion of 'quality' then became favoured as a most convenient caption under which the Conservatives could implement their second wave of managerial reforms in the late 1980s. The idea of providing a quality service could at the same time serve to reassure an anxious public, boost the morale of service providers, and allow government to increase its control over professional groups by setting, monitoring and evaluating performance against quality targets.[27]

Under the Conservatives, the notion of quality was developed by analogy with a business providing a good product to its customers. The ideology of quality was directly imported from the commercial world, where it was expressed, for example, in the British Standard 5750 quality mark and in the school of 'total quality management' (TQM). In industry, TQM is a means by which management tries to motivate the whole work-force behind its aim to deliver products to a particular specification. It was widely believed that the application of private sector management techniques and disciplines to the NHS could improve the quality of the product. Thus the White Papers *Working for Patients* (1989) and *Competing for Quality* (1991) initiated and accelerated the drive towards markets and quasi-markets in the health service, in the belief that an improvement in quality would follow.

Correspondingly, neoliberal doctrine encouraged us to see the producer–consumer relationship as the standard way of relating to one another. As far as health was concerned, this meant that individuals should learn to see themselves as consumers rather than as patients. They should no longer be content to be the grateful beneficiaries of professional benevolence, but rather they should insist on their rights. Thus, in its late 1980s/early 1990s guise, 'quality' was the emblem under which a new consumer-oriented NHS was urged upon us. John Major's *Patients' Charter* promised a health service that would be quicker, more responsive and easier to complain about when things went wrong.

Doctors did not on the whole welcome the advent of consumerism in medicine. Moreover, it was easy to caricature this type of quality as amounting to little more than the customer's freedom to comment on the choice of decor in the hospital ward. However, under New Labour the notion of quality took on a deeper meaning. Quality moved well beyond the domain of economics and consumer choice into the heartlands of clinical practice. The stated objective of New Labour is to '*ensure that quality of care becomes the driving force for the development of health services in England*'.[28] The government is doing this by moving beyond the Conservative party's attempt to control medical professionals through management and management techniques. New Labour is intent on controlling medical practice from within professional groups themselves by implementing a new culture of clinical governance.

The crucial organisational unit within which the new culture will be embedded is the PCG/PCT. Liam Donaldson comments:

> *There is little doubt that the development of primary care groups and trusts, with clear corporate goals and objectives directed towards quality improvement and the development of their staff, will be the keys to the success of clinical governance in primary care.*[25]

The Chief Executive and Board of a PCG/PCT have a statutory duty with regard to the implementation of clinical governance. This involves establishing leadership, accountability and working arrangements, formulating and agreeing a development plan and establishing a reporting arrangement for clinical governance within board and annual reports. Since six or seven of the 11 or 12 members of PCG boards are usually GPs, it is the representatives of the professions themselves, elected by their peers, who are set up to be responsible for ensuring that clinical governance is put in place. It will be doctors themselves who are challenging clinical autonomy in the name of clinical governance.

This represents a very considerable change in culture. The doctors and nurses of the future will not typically work in single-handed or small practices, but rather they will be members of PCGs or PCTs with perhaps up to 50 doctors. They may be partners or salaried employees, and their loyalty will be increasingly less towards their own professional group, and increasingly more towards the Board of their own group or trust. It is this group to which the new GP will be financially and clinically accountable. Doctors who place a high value on professional autonomy will not find this an easy cultural shift.

Comparison with a similar group: the teaching profession

To gain some sense of the possible impact of modernisation on doctors as a profession, it is worth considering a parallel with the teaching profession. Certainly teachers do not undertake the same long period of training, nor do they enjoy the same social status and income as GPs. However, like doctors, they are paid out of public funds, and they work in a field which has been the subject of intense political interest in recent years. Moreover, teachers are higher up the political agenda. In a 'modern' context, the first political priority is 'education, education, education'. To see where GPs may be in the future, it is worth casting a sideways glance to see where teachers are now.

There has been a revolution in the classroom during the last decade. Not so long ago, teachers had a high degree of control over what and how they taught, headteachers had a high degree of control over their staff and pupils, and local education authorities controlled finance and many policy areas. By contrast, parents were kept firmly at the school gate, governors were shadowy figures whom no one knew and who exercised little real power, and voluntary and business organisations were mostly irrelevant to the life of the school.

Today, teachers must teach in accordance with nationally developed curricula. In primary schools, even the way in which they teach is prescribed by government in sensitive curriculum areas, such as literacy. There is increasing pressure from government to link teachers' pay with the performance of their pupils in national tests. Headteachers are now much more accountable to their governors, and the powers of local authorities are being progressively reduced. School governors, by contrast, now have responsibility for school finance and many policy areas that were previously controlled by the local authority. Parents are welcomed into the classroom to work alongside teachers as helpers. The quality of the school's performance is monitored by nationally assessed tests and by five-yearly OFSTED inspections which deliver public reports. In addition, local businesses and voluntary organisations (e.g. churches) are welcomed into partnership with some schools, and may even be invited to take over the management of 'failing' schools.

The effects of these massive changes include the following:

- increased national control over the delivery and quality of education
- a considerable reduction in the autonomy of teachers
- some increases in the powers of parents
- increases in the possibility of local communities 'owning' their schools, and of partnerships with other local organisations.

By analogy, we might expect – and indeed are already beginning to see – the following parallel changes in the arena of health:

- increased national control over the delivery and quality of primary care
- a reduction in the autonomy of GPs
- some increases in the powers of patients
- increased opportunities for local communities to own their primary care groups or trusts.

It is only fair to say that, whatever its impact on educational standards (and the jury is still out on this one), modernisation has had some significant downsides as far as the teaching profession is concerned. Teachers routinely complain of too fast a rate of change, a proliferation of targets, too much documentation, too much emphasis on quantitative assessment, reduced professional self-esteem, long working hours and inadequate recognition. It remains to be seen whether GPs, with their stronger professional muscle, can avoid similar downsides themselves.

The changing role of the GP

The values of New Labour challenge the traditional values of the GP. The theme of modernisation is being powerfully played out across a range of different areas of life, of which primary healthcare is just one. A set of modern structures (most notably the PCG/PCT), a modern ideology (quality) and a modern implementation method (clinical governance) are already in place. All of these make it likely that being a 'new GP' will feel quite different.

Of course it would be easy to feel nostalgic for an earlier golden era.[29] Doctors in this country have until now enjoyed a high and distinctive level of social status and a good deal of control over their own practice. It is natural for them to want to hold on to this as far as possible. However, in the era of 'modernisation', some of this is going to change. The single-handed practitioner will give way to the partner or, more likely, employee in a primary care trust. Collaboration will assume a higher value than autonomy, and there will be more accountability and more quality control. There could be some blurring of roles with other health service groups, most notably with nurses, although whether nurses will want to take on the tyes of professional responsibilities so far shouldered only by GPs remains to be seen. This may not seem like a very enticing prospect.

However, there are positive opportunities, too. In a major article at the start of the new millennium, Chancellor Gordon Brown encouraged the nation *'not to fear change but to embrace it'*.[30] He proceeded to set out a 'Third Way' vision of civic society, transcending the communitarianism of the left and the individualism of the right.

Significantly, as his primary example of an institution which expressed his notion of 'civic society', he chose the National Health Service. Quoting Jonathan Sacks' *Politics of Hope*,[31] Brown went on to offer a vision of a *covenant-based* society in which a common purpose among different people is established through a commitment to shared values. His choice of the NHS was not accidental. In a pluralistic, post-Christian society the NHS does indeed offer one of the few national institutions around which people unite. Those who have significant roles within it therefore have special opportunities for wider civic leadership.

The Green Paper entitled *Our Healthier Nation*[32] and the subsequent White Paper, *Saving Lives*,[1] both argue for a three-way contract or partnership (or what might better, following Sacks and Brown, be called covenant) for improving the nation's health. This sets out responsibilities for individuals, for government and for local communities. At a community level, health authorities and PCGs/PCTs will have the major responsibility for programmes of health improvement. Doctors may now have opportunities which extend well beyond the medical care of individual patients. Working in partnership with NHS colleagues, Social Services, local councils, schools and other voluntary groups, they have the opportunity to play a leading role in improving the health and well-being of a local population.

This may prove too grand a vision and involve too rapid a pace of change. However, if the professional groups can shape and manage the vision, there is a real chance of creating a new and vibrant professional identity. As we have argued elsewhere,[33] the notion of covenant is central to the doctor–patient relationship. What is needed now is some very careful thinking about how this notion might be extended to cater for the wider expectations that are being placed upon doctors by New Labour. The ethic of 'modernisation' calls for a new professional identity, centred now not on the privilege of self-regulation, nor even on exclusive duties to individual patients, but on a wider set of covenant responsibilities and civic service.

Summary points

- Modernisation is a sociological term which traditionally described the evolution of primitive societies to industrialised societies.
- The term has been given particular content by the politicians of the Third Way.
- The Third Way – the political ideology of New Labour and other centre-left governments – is a response to new global conditions.
- It is an attempt to transcend old-style socialism and the neoliberalism of recent Conservative governments.
- The core values of the Third Way include equality and protection of the vulnerable, as well as 'no rights without responsibilities'.
- Primary care trusts and clinical governance represent the NHS embodiment of Third Way modernisation.
- The medical profession can learn from the impact of modernisation on the teaching profession.
- The ethic of modernisation calls for a new professional identity based less on the privilege of self-regulation and the duty to individual patients, and more on a wider set of covenanted relationships and civic service.

References

1   Secretary of State for Health (1999) *Saving Lives: Our Healthier Nation*. HMSO, London.

2   Minister for the Cabinet Office (1999) *Modernising Government*. HMSO, London.

3   Giddens A (1999) *The Third Way: The Renewal of Social Democracy*. Polity, Cambridge.

4   The general conditions asserted throughout Giddens A (1999) *The Third Way: The Renewal of Social Democracy*. Polity, Cambridge.

5   See, for example, Leadbeater C (1999) *Living on Thin Air: The New Economy*. Penguin, Harmondsworth.

6   The moderate socialism of Western European left-wing parties (including the UK Labour party) was discredited by the inability of its policies of economic management to deal with the inflationary crisis of the late 1970s. The Communistic forms of socialism prevalent in Eastern Europe were defeated in 1989, both in reality and symbolically, with the fall of the Berlin Wall.

7   The sociologist George Ritzer has famously interpreted this in terms of the 'McDonaldization' of many aspects of society, including education, work, healthcare, travel,

politics and the family. See Ritzer G (1996) *The McDonaldization of Society*. Pine Forge Press, CA.

8   Perhaps most significantly, the increasing levels of female participation in the work-force. The Council of Churches for Britain and Ireland (1997) *Unemployment and the Future of Work* (CCBI, London) comments that 'The fact that women as well as men now expect to take part in paid work is itself a change in the nature of work and society of immense significance. It is at least as important and challenging as the development of new technology. ... The industrial revolution brought about a very sharp distinction between the work that men and women do. ... In a post-industrial society, if that is the right term to describe the patterns of life and work now emerging, men and women may again see their tasks as, in many if not all respects, the same.' Women accounted for only 25% of those entering the medical profession in the 1960s, but have represented around 50% of medical graduates for most of the 1990s (*see* chapter by Isobel Allen in Harrison J and van Zwanenberg T (eds) (1998) *GP Tomorrow*. Radcliffe Medical Press, Oxford, 143–53).

9   For a discussion of the phenomenon of globalisation, see Baylis J and Smith S (eds) (1998) *The Globalization of World Politics*. Oxford University Press, Oxford. Also Tomlinson J (1999) *Globalization and Culture*. Polity, Cambridge. 'Globalisation' is succinctly defined by Baylis and Smith as 'the process of increasing connectedness between societies such that events in one part of the world more and more have effects on people and societies far away. A globalised world is one in which political, economic, cultural and social events become more and more interconnected.'

10 See, for example, the argument of one of Blair's favourite gurus: Leadbeater C (1999) *Living on Thin Air: The New Economy*. Penguin, Harmondsworth.

11 Selbourne D (1999) All that is solid melts into Blair. *The Times*. 30 December.

12 Giddens A (1999) *The Third Way: The Renewal of Social Democracy*. Polity, Cambridge.

13 For a full treatment, see Aviner S and de-Shalit A (eds) (1992) *Communitarianism and Individualism*. Oxford University Press, Oxford. See also Bell D (1993) *Communitarianism and its Critics*. Clarendon Press, Oxford.

14 See further discussion of 'conservatism' in Ashford N and Davies S (eds) (1991) *A Dictionary of Conservative and Libertarian Thought*. Routledge, London.

15 Aviner S and de-Shalit A (1992), *op. cit.*

16 See discussion of 'modernisation' in Bealey F (1999) *The Blackwell Dictionary of Political Science*. Basil Blackwell, Oxford. Compare with Giddens A (2000) *The Third Way and its Critics*. Polity, Cambridge: 'Modernisation here means reforming social institutions to meet the demands of a globalising information order. It is certainly not to be identified solely with economic development.'

17 Ashford and Davies (1991)[14] entry on 'neoliberalism'.

18 *New Shorter Oxford English Dictionary* (1993). Clarendon, Oxford. See also entry on 'pluralism' in Bealey F (1999).[16]

19 *New Shorter Oxford English Dictionary*. See also entry on 'socialism' in Bealey (1999).[16] Bealey comments that 'There is a divide among socialists about how much industry ought

to be publicly owned. Communists would say all of it; many socialists would go no further than public utilities such as gas and water.'

20   Theakston K (1999) In: G Taylor (ed.) *The Impact of New Labour.* Macmillan, London.

21   Blair T (1996) *New Britain: My Vision of a Young Country.* New Statesman, London.

22   Minister for the Cabinet Office (1999) *Modernising Government.* HMSO, London. See also Meads G and Ashcroft J (2000) *Relationships in the NHS.* Royal Society of Medicine Press, London and Blair T (1999) Foreword. In: T Coffy, G Boersma, L Smith and P Wallace (eds) *Visions of Primary Care.* New Health Network, London.

23   http://www.number-10.gov.uk/default.asp?PageId=757

24   Meads G and Ashcroft J (2000) *Relationships in the NHS.* Royal Society of Medicine Press, London.

25   Donaldson L (2000) In: T van Zwanenberg and J Harrison (ed.) *Clinical Governance in Primary Care.* Radcliffe Medical Press, Oxford.

26   Koch H (1991) Buying and selling high-quality health care. In: P Spurgeon (ed.) *The Changing Face of the National Health Service in the 1990s.* Longman, Harlow.

27   See, for example, Harrison S and Politt C (1994) *Controlling Health Professionals.* Open University Press, Buckingham.

28   NHS Executive (1998) *Quality in the New NHS.* Department of Health, Wetherby.

29   See, for example, Morrell D (1998) The NHS's 50th Anniversary. *BMJ.* **317**: 40–45, who locates the golden age of the GP in the late 1970s and early 1980s.

30   Brown G (2000) *The Times.* 10 January.

31   Sacks J (1997) *The Politics of Hope.* Cape, London.

32   Secretary of State for Health (1998) *Our Healthier Nation: A Contract for Health.* HMSO, London.

33   Harrison J and Innes R (1997) *Medical Vocation and Generation X.* Grove, Cambridge.

PART 2

The features of modernisation

CHAPTER FIVE

Triage and its application to *NHS Direct* and walk-in centres

Kevin McKenna

There is no telling what people might find out once they felt free to ask whatever they wanted to.

Joseph Heller

This chapter describes the basis of triage and how it is being used in *NHS Direct* and walk-in centres. Triage enables patients to be prioritised and 'signposted' to the appropriate level of care.

Managing demand

The open-ended GP Contract meant that general practitioners used to be the key 24-hour-a-day filter in the process of managed care.* From 1948, the model shown in Figure 5.1 has applied, and demonstrates the 'triage gateway' to NHS services being managed by the GP.

---

*Managed care is defined as 'the arrangement whereby an organisation assumes responsibility for all necessary healthcare for an individual in exchange for fixed payment'.

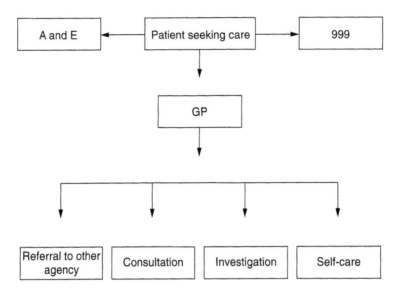

Figure 5.1   The 'triage gateway' to NHS services.

With an expansion in the services offered, social changes and an increasing workload, it is hardly surprising that the GP filter became overloaded. The consequent overflow of patients, generally acknowledged to be presenting with conditions appropriate to primary care, then caused significant problems in the other two traditional gateways to the NHS, namely the Accident and Emergency (A and E) departments and the ambulance services.[1]

Modernisation of the NHS is designed to enhance the 'supply side' of healthcare provision by increasing access to services and making them more sensitive to the needs of patients.[2] Redesigning so-called 'patient-friendly' pathways of access, which simultaneously offer advice and information, could not only improve the delivery of care, but might also manage demand better by enabling patients to help themselves. It is argued that such an increase in patients' abilities with regard to self-care would create 'headroom' in the system for the professionals, who are under pressure. However, the professionals would have to adapt their practice accordingly.

Telephone triage using computer decision support systems (CDSS) was developed in the USA, and is currently being adopted all over the world as a tool for managing demand. The systems in use vary in their structure (the way they are intended to work) and performance (how successful they are). At the heart of the design of all of the systems is the ability to separate safely those patients who require the intervention of a health professional from those who do not.

In addition, the systems can map care pathways in a way that could reduce some of the variation in access to services. This variation is a major issue for the government. For example, there is a fourfold difference in admission rates for patients over 75 years of age, and there is even considerable variability in home-visiting rates in primary care.[3]

Triage and access

The NHS can seem like a maze, even for those who work in it. Patients could be forgiven for sometimes stumbling into services where they are considered to be 'inappropriate attenders'. This mishap is then compounded by poor communication within the NHS, resulting in the same question being asked and recorded over and over again before the patient eventually finds the correct pathway to the appropriate service. In these circumstances, access to care may depend more on the mood of staff or the forcefulness of the patient than on the clinical priority of the presenting problem.

Thus an ability to prioritise patients who use the service can be seen as critical to the development of a consistent 'needs-led' service. Moreover, a clinically prioritised triage 'entry system', which incorporates a health information service, a language line (offering different languages) and Minicom facilities (for the deaf), would clearly enable and empower certain groups who currently find it difficult to obtain the relevant healthcare. In this way the application of new technology could provide more equitable access to services.

Triage is the process of prioritising. It involves placing a range of issues, as presented to the individual responsible for their resolution, in order of importance. The term has its origin in French agriculture, where it was used to describe the sorting of livestock at market. It was first used in a medical context by Baron Dominique Larry, when he was appointed as Napoleon's Surgeon General and developed the '*Hôpital de triage*'. These field hospitals sorted casualties into three categories, so that battlefield surgeons could focus their attention on those individuals who were most likely to benefit from their intervention (*see* Table 5.1). A similar approach to triage is used by modern-day Forward Medical Aid Units (FMAUs) in the context of major disasters and war.

Telephone triage

Nurses who use telephone triage are known to be as effective as doctors in determining whether, when and where a patient needs further assessment by their general practitioner.[4] In contrast, general practitioners and casualty staff are rarely taught the art of telephone consultation,[5] and may therefore be more likely to make mistakes when responding to

Table 5.1 Battlefield triage

Category	Assessment	Action
A	Life-threatening injury where immediate medical intervention will make a difference	Resuscitate and treat immediately
B	Minor injury where immediate medical intervention is not imperative	Give first aid and reassess later
C	(Death or) so severe an injury that immediate medical intervention is unlikely to make any difference	Give first aid only and reassess later

patients on the phone. Without the nuances of body language, clinicians may struggle to assess clinical problems accurately. It then becomes difficult to prioritise them safely. The resultant anxiety caused by consulting by telephone, and the inability to make a satisfactory assessment, may lead to unnecessary face-to-face consultations, to the inconvenience of both doctor and patient.

However, over-confidence among clinicians about their ability to triage increases clinical risk by inappropriately advising self-care when a face-to-face consultation is required. For example, it is known that there is wide variation between general prac- titioners in the proportion of contacts managed by telephone advice alone rather than by face-to-face consultation, ranging from 10% to 65%, with a mean of 38%.[6] If patients are to be given self-care advice over the telephone as part of a demand-management strategy, consistency in approach is essential.

Clinical assessment by telephone requires subtle techniques which are not necessarily applicable in face-to-face consultations. For example, telephone assessment of abdominal pain must exclude the possibility of peritonism if a face-to-face consultation is to be avoided. Peritoneal irritation can be excluded by asking the patient to stand up on their toes and rock back sharply on to their heels. If this movement exacerbates the abdominal pain, peritonism cannot be excluded and the patient should be seen.[7]

Decision-supported triage

The idea of CDSS is not new. Most doctors began their careers as house officers with a dog-eared *aide-mémoire* on emergency care in their white-coat pockets. With the advent of the computer there has been a step change in the power, speed and process of decision support.

There are three telephone triage systems in use in the NHS (*see* Box 5.1). They differ in their logic structure (the theoretical basis on which they work), sorting characteristics (the proportion of patients allocated to the different categories) and risk management profiles (the likelihood of generating inappropriate advice).

Recent publications from North America have elaborated on the risks associated with the protocol and cognitive models of telephone triage.[8] Given their structure, it is not sur- prising that the outcomes obtained with these two models are more variable than those obtained with the algorithmic model.[9] The algorithmic system still requires considerable clinical expertise from the nurse in taking a history, and it is more time consuming and thus more costly than the other models.

The NHS has to assess the cost-effectiveness of the three models in the context of the 'whole system'. For example, it could be more cost-effective to use an expensive system with low risk and better sorting in order to reduce the pressure on other parts of the NHS and thereby make economies. Equally, it could be more cost-effective to use a cheaper system and to accept lower standards of sorting. Whichever system is adopted, perform- ance depends as much on the selection, training and monitoring of the staff who use it as it does on the nature of the system itself.

Box 5.1:   **Triage models used by *NHS Direct***

The cognitive model
The nurse is prompted to ask relevant questions for any given clinical presentation. At the end of the process, the nurse collates the information and *intuitively* decides from a fixed list of alternatives (Accident and Emergency, self-care, urgent GP care, etc.) which is the most appropriate outcome. The system makes no recommendation about the most suitable outcome.

The protocol model
This model is more structured. Questions to identify or exclude serious problems are asked at the beginning, and each subsequent question is targeted at conditions of lesser severity. Using this hierarchical approach a mere three questions may result in an emergency ambulance for a patient with chest pain, six questions in attendance at Accident and Emergency, four in a GP appointment and eight in self-care. Although the nurse can override the system, the software recommends both the timing and nature of intervention required.

The algorithmic model
This system is like the game of '20 questions', and is based on a sequence of questions with yes/no answers. This 'binary branch logic' system takes into account the prevalence and severity of serious conditions that might be associated with the presenting symptom, and assesses the risk associated with missing that condition (e.g. high risk for meningitis, low risk for migraine). Using this mathematical model, a logic tree is established for each symptom, which systematically excludes conditions in decreasing order of severity. Ultimately it reaches a point where a condition cannot be excluded. The system then recommends the nature and timing of intervention required.

Rather than opting for any of the current systems, the government has chosen to define requirements, and to invite suppliers to tender against these. It is anticipated that the system will be able to be used in face-to-face settings, and be networked on a national basis to establish a virtual call centre.

The politics of *NHS Direct*

NHS Direct and walk-in centres, rather like 'sex and violence', have generated a good deal of sometimes heated debate, particularly when paired as discussion topics. Many general practitioners have yet to see or believe in their value as management tools. Some fear that they may cause a breakdown in professional relationships between general practitioners and their patients, loss of control, and a consumer-driven workload that is not matched by resources. Yet the Department of Health report on emergency services in the community indicated that considerable strain, particularly out of hours, was being put on Accident and Emergency departments and the ambulance services.[10] The report concluded that many of these patients would be better dealt with in primary care, thereby enabling the performance standards of the acute services to be improved.

The irony of the situation was that many patients were using these services inappropriately because primary care itself was under great strain. Thus patients were overflowing into the only other points of access to NHS services.

The incoming Labour administration continued with plans which had been considered by the outgoing Conservative government, for a nurse-led health helpline (*NHS Direct*) that might alleviate some of the pressure on the acute services. Previous experience in Health Maintenance Organisations (HMOs) in the USA indicated that helplines could be used cost-effectively as demand management tools. They also appeared to produce high levels of patient satisfaction.

NHS Direct seemed to offer the core of a programme which, by providing information, could educate and empower patients and bring services closer to their homes. With a triage system (sometimes called a 'platform' in the jargon) incorporated, it offered an opportunity to cut across many of the established professional barriers. It might thus facilitate modernisation of and better communication within the wider NHS.

Although *NHS Direct* started as a pilot development, ministers made it clear that the pilot was all about the 'how?' rather than the 'whether?'. *NHS Direct* was to be developed nation-wide. The Sheffield evaluation[11] reinforced the political belief in high levels of patient satisfaction, and what had at first seemed to be a marginal development soon became a key pillar in the process of NHS modernisation. Senior politicians were behind it, and complete coverage of England was promised by the end of the year 2000.

General practitioners and other health professionals found the scale and rate of development difficult to accept. There was fierce criticism of the lack of evidence of cost-effectiveness, given the constraints on other areas of NHS spending. The potential impact on other services, which were already experiencing difficulty in recruiting nurses, was highlighted as another important issue that had apparently not been considered by the government.

NHS Direct developments

The initial evaluation of *NHS Direct* concentrated on three pilot sites in Tyneside, Lancashire and Buckinghamshire. Successive waves of pilot sites, usually based in ambulance trusts as the host organisation, quickly evolved during 1998 and 1999. Emphasis was placed on partnership working between those 'stakeholders' in the management structures who might be most affected. Each pilot site was thus based on a management structure including a Director of Nursing, a Medical Director, a Project Manager and a Call Centre Manager, each of whom was answerable to the Chief Executive of the parent trust.

It was probably naive to think that an ambulance trust's expertise in communications equipped it to run a complex call centre staffed by nurses. The disparate interests and cultures involved meant that there was often difficulty in achieving consensus.

The initial rate of uptake by the public was low and proportional to local publicity,[11] but early experience confirmed the findings from elsewhere (*see* Box 5.2).

Box 5.2:   Early experience of *NHS Direct*

By December 1998:

- 60 000 calls had been taken nation-wide
- four million people were covered
- there was a staff complement of 22.5 whole-time-equivalent nurses and 27 operators
- the pattern of demand was similar to that seen in out-of-hours primary care
- 25% of calls related to the under-5-years age group
- the range and pattern of illness was the same as in conventional primary care.

The second wave of pilot sites was invited to consider the potential for integrating services, including, for example, the triage of:

- GP and dental out-of-hours calls
- Category 'C' (low-priority) calls to the ambulance service
- mental health services' calls
- Social Services' calls.

A range of other projects (e.g. chronic disease management systems) was also considered. A variety of points of access to *NHS Direct*, including digital television and email services, was promised by the end of the year 2000.[12] A remote link with *NHS Direct*, or being co-located on the same site, was a prerequisite for the NHS walk-in centres. *NHS Direct* information points are eventually to be established in public places such as libraries, schools and shopping centres.

Key to the success of *NHS Direct* is the provision of accurate information on health topics, and the Health Information Service is being incorporated into *NHS Direct* during the year 2000. There are allegedly 100 000 health-related sites on the Internet, and their number is probably a reflection of their popularity with patients. But how can a patient know if the advice given is valid? In November 1999, the Secretary of State launched the *NHS Direct* website, and the *NHS Direct* self-care guidebook. The website provides links to other approved sites. The advice given is consistent with the other *NHS Direct* systems (platforms) and is based either on consensus in the UK or on evidence. The website received 1.5 million visitors ('hits') on its first day of operation, and is currently contacted over 100 000 times daily.

NHS Direct evaluation

An independent evaluation of *NHS Direct* was commissioned from the University of Sheffield. However, the pace of development and extension of sites, the dramatic increase in use of the service at the end of the evaluation period, and rapid changes in the structure of the organisation itself have all tended to make the results of the study less relevant than was anticipated. In particular, there has been no assessment of the actual clinical outcomes resulting from the nurses' advice. When comparing the systems, evaluation has shown that the algorithm model takes significantly longer to triage calls than the other two systems, but that patient satisfaction levels are also significantly higher. There were marked differences in the systems' sorting of patients (e.g. in the proportions of patients advised to attend Accident and Emergency departments) (*see* Table 5.2).

Each of the systems' sorting characteristics was tested by presenting them with 120 simulated calls, derived from calls to three ambulance services that had been classed as lowest priority. In each real case the patient had been taken to hospital by ambulance but not admitted. Centramax (protocol system) and the Telephone Advice System (cognitive system) both directed 44% of these simulated calls to an urgent Accident and Emergency attendance, whereas Personal Health Adviser (algorithm system) directed only 23% to an urgent Accident and Emergency attendance. Thus it appears that the differences are due primarily to the way in which urgent calls are handled (by the systems), and not to differences in the types of calls being made to each site.[11]

Because the initial volume of calls was low, when compared to the very large volume received by existing services, the evaluation has been limited in its conclusions. *NHS Direct* is clinically safe, and the major concern that it might drive up demand from the worried well has not been confirmed.[11] However, one critical question remains unanswered. Is it a cost-effective management tool?

> *If it turns out to be the case that* NHS Direct *has provided easier and faster advice and information, and has improved access to appropriate health care for those who need it, then the fact that this will have been achieved without increasing overall demand is clearly an encouraging and positive finding. Placed alongside the earlier evidence of very high caller satisfaction with the service, these findings taken together suggest that* NHS Direct *may be beginning to achieve the policy objectives for which it was designed.*[11]

Table 5.2   Percentage of callers advised to attend Accident and Emergency (A and E) departments*

System type	System make	Percentage advised to attend A and E departments
Algorithm	Personal Health Adviser (PHA), Access Health UK	9
Protocol	Centramax, HBOC UK	21
Cognitive	Telephone Advice System (TAS), Plain Software	36

*Other factors, such as the nurses being attached to the A and E department at the TAS site, mean that the figures need to be interpreted with caution.

NHS Direct and NHS Net

A major future challenge will be to ensure that the advice given to patients by *NHS Direct* is linked to their clinical record and available to the patient's general practitioner when they see them. Failure to achieve this will ultimately cause difficulties for patients and considerable irritation for the doctors and nurses responsible for their continuing care.

If *NHS Direct* is to form part of a coherent NHS framework for patient care, it is vital that the information it handles:

- is valid and evidence based
- can be transferred easily between providers
- can be transferred confidentially.

Current electronic communication systems in the NHS are poor. The NHS Net, which is the likely conduit for such data transfer, has yet to be developed to a point where it would engender confidence among NHS staff that it could deliver the above standards. The NHS messaging service has limitations, and there are concerns about the security and technology of NHS Net. As is often the case with what is perceived to be flawed technology, human frailty and organisations are more often the real problem.

It is vital that the electronic 'firewall' between NHS Net and the Internet is secure. However, the security which will enable clinical patient information to flow confidentially between providers will depend more on satisfactory encryption procedures, and the internal security arrangements of NHS organisations, than on the firewall itself. One million people work in the NHS, and the proportion of hackers is probably no lower than in the rest of the population.

Adequate security and guaranteed performance from providers is simply not possible on the Internet itself, and a separate NHS network is therefore essential. However, NHS organisations must develop adequate address-book services that are continuously updated for any email system to succeed. Most of the current NHS messaging difficulties are actually caused by organisations failing to provide up-to-date databases. Developing and sustaining these, although difficult to achieve, is a prerequisite for 'connectivity' in the NHS and thus for modernisation.

Walk-in centres and *NHS Direct*

The government recognised that certain groups in the population, notably urban commuters, were experiencing difficulty in gaining access to primary care services. For people working away from their homes, the office hours of general practice may prove an obstacle to seeking care. As noted in other chapters, the 24-hour consumer culture is at variance with the traditional timetables of morning and evening surgery.

Furthermore, there had been a growth in GP out-of-hours co-operatives, which were popular with patients previously used to the conventional model of out-of-hours care.[12,13]

Although doctors and patients recognised that conventional practice-based primary care was valuable in terms of continuity, patients seemed quite happy to use alternative services for acute problems.

In April 1999, the Prime Minister announced the programme for the development of walk-in centres. Their brief was to offer, on a drop-in basis, minor treatments, health information and self-help advice to the public. They were to be managed by an established NHS body or GP co-operative. In particular, they were to be sited in a demonstrably convenient location to enable easy access, and to operate at times when conventional primary care services were normally unavailable.

The walk-in centres were to complement – not replace – conventional GP services, and patients who were not registered with a doctor were to be encouraged to register.[12] The walk-in centres would often be linked to the *NHS Direct* triage system (platform) and offer the same information and advice. They might be on the same site as a GP co-operative or minor injuries unit, and they might be home to a range of clinical and associated services.

By using the *NHS Direct* triage platform in the walk-in centres, the identical process of validated triage could be assured. Without it, patients who were dissatisfied with advice given by *NHS Direct* might bypass *NHS Direct* and present at a walk-in centre for a 'second opinion'. As over 94% of the population have access to a telephone, it would seem more likely that patients would either visit the website, read the book or telephone for advice from their own home, rather than travel to a walk-in centre.

The future

Work is currently in progress on Tyneside using the *NHS Direct* triage platform at the front of an Accident and Emergency department. Initial evaluation suggests that the outcome is almost identical to that achieved using the platform on the telephone, and patient satisfaction is equally high (Urgent Needs Assessment Service, North Tyneside District General Hospital, North Tyneside, Tyne and Wear, unpublished data). If these results are confirmed, then it is possible that the NHS, at least out of hours, could provide patients who are seeking acute care with a consistent triage pathway into services at all points of access.

General practitioners are rightly apprehensive about work being 'dumped' on them from other sectors in the NHS, but they may be prepared to consider such a model if a validated triage platform can ensure that they see only an appropriate mix of patients. If that triage platform can also safely guide a significant proportion of patients, unseen, to self-care, the incessant growth in workload might be arrested.

There is financial logic, as well as convenience for patients, in co-locating out-of-hours primary care centres, minor injury units, walk-in centres, dental units, and so on. Economies of scale, staff integration and more efficient service provision are attractive to politicians and primary care managers alike.

Implications for the new GP

The advent of sophisticated triage platforms, operated by nurses at access points to acute care, may have a profound impact on the way in which NHS services are used. At best, they offer coherent and consistent advice and faster access for patients to what they need. At worst, they might damage doctor–patient relationships and hinder effective long-term care. If a nurse and a decision support system can safely triage patients to appropriate levels of care more cheaply than a general practitioner, a redefinition of roles becomes inevitable. Such developments in the 'Information Age' are understandably unsettling, and some of the resistance to and scepticism about *NHS Direct* may arise from apprehension about the impact of information technology on the future role and function of the general practitioner.

The frenetic pace of development of *NHS Direct* and the absence of validated UK data on outcomes of the triage process have also unsettled general practitioners. The pace of development will slow down. For one thing, the pool of nurses (currently around 600) needed to staff the call centres is not immediately available. Indeed, careful management is required to prevent recruitment to *NHS Direct* undermining other key NHS services.

Decision support has been considered here in the context of nurse-operated triage. However, general practitioners are familiar with Prodigy. Moreover, the 'utilisation management tools' currently in use in the USA will surely make their appearance here in due course. These tools help clinicians to define the level and type of care that a patient requires for any given condition. In hospitals, for example, they are used to allocate patients to the category of bed that is most suitable at any given time.

The future role of *NHS Direct* will become clearer over time. Could it, for example, become the 'front end' of all services? Given the volume of calls involved, this seems unlikely, but its greater deployment in primary care is inevitable. Indeed, some general practitioners are already looking to use *NHS Direct* to triage their daytime calls, and are offering access to their appointment books as soon as suitable IT links can be established.

In conclusion, general practitioners will continue to be involved in the vast majority of patient care in the NHS. In the USA the two most favoured management technologies, namely decision support and managed care, have been largely driven by the desire to contain costs. This has felt uncomfortable for physicians. In the UK there is the opportunity to define the structure and use of both around the principles of quality and governance. The systems themselves will shape many pathways of care, and will influence how medicine is practised in this country. The new GP will need to consider how he or she can contribute to influencing the shape and development of these systems.

Summary points

- Triage is the process of prioritising, which was first used in a medical context in military field hospitals to sort the casualties of war.
- Telephone triage using computer decision support systems (CDSS) was developed in the USA, and is currently being adopted world-wide as a tool for managing demand.
- There are different systems available, but all of them are designed to separate safely those patients who require the intervention of a health professional from those who do not.
- *NHS Direct* simultaneously offers advice and information, and may not only improve access to care, but might also manage demand better by enabling patients to help themselves.
- An increase in self-care might create 'headroom' for the professionals who are currently under pressure.
- Walk-in centres are using the identical triage system (platform) in a face-to-face setting.
- The *NHS Direct* triage platform could become the 'front end' of all points of access for out-of-hours care – telephone helpline, Accident and Emergency, walk-in centres and GP out-of-hours services.
- *NHS Direct* prioritises and 'signposts' patients to the appropriate level of care. It does not diagnose.

References

1 Nicholl J, Turner J and Pickin M (1998) *A Review of Evidence for the Provision of Emergency Services*. Medical Care Research Unit, University of Sheffield, Sheffield.

2 Department of Health (1997) *The New NHS: Modern, Dependable*. The Stationery Office, London.

3 Department of Health (1999) *Shaping the Future NHS. Long-Term Planning for Hospitals and Related Services. Consultation Document on the Findings of the National Beds Inquiry*. Department of Health, London; website www.doh.gov.uk/nationalbeds.htm

4 Lattimer V, George S, Thompson F *et al.* (1998) Safety and effectiveness of nurse telephone consultations in out-of-hours primary care: randomised controlled trial (the South Wiltshire Out-of-Hours Project (SWOOP) Group). *BMJ.* **317**: 1054–9.

5 Evans RJ, McCabe M, Allen H, Rainer T and Richmond PW (1993) Telephone advice in the Accident and Emergency department: a survey of current practice. *Arch Emerg Med.* **10**: 216–19.

6 Jessop I, Beck I, Hollins L, Shipman C, Reynolds M and Dale J (1997) Changing the pattern out of hours: a survey of GP co-operatives. *BMJ.* **314**: 199–200.

7 Personal Health Adviser, Access Health UK *Abdominal Pain Assessment Algorithm*. Personal Health Adviser, Access Health UK.

8   Wachter DA, Brillman JC, Lewis J and Sapien RE (1999) Pediatric telephone triage protocols: standardized decision-making or a false sense of security? *Ann Emerg Med.* **33**: 388–94.

9   Brillman JC, Doezema D, Tandberg D *et al.* (1996) Triage: limitations in predicting need for emergency care and hospital admission. *Ann Emerg Med.* **27**: 493–500.

10   Department of Health (1997) *Developing Emergency Services in the Community. The Final Report.* Department of Health, London.

11   Munro J, Nicholl J, O'Cathain A and Knowles E (2000) *Evaluation of* NHS Direct. Medical Care Research Unit, University of Sheffield, Sheffield.

12   Department of Health (1999) *NHS Primary Care Walk-in Centres.* Department of Health, London.

13   Hallam L and Henthorne K (1999) *Providing Out-of-Hours Primary Care in Northumberland: an Evaluation of the Development, Operations and Impact of the Northumberland Out-of-Hours Co-operative.* National Primary Care Research and Development Centre, University of Manchester, Manchester.

CHAPTER SIX

Continuing professional development

Stephen Sylvester

If the license to practise meant the completion of his education, how sad would it be for the practitioner, how distressing to his patients.

Sir William Osler

Continuing professional development is a process of lifelong learning for all individuals and teams which meets the needs of patients and delivers the health outcomes and health-care priorities of the NHS and which enables professionals to expand and fulfil their potential.

A First-Class Service: Quality in the New NHS[1]

This chapter describes a new approach to continuing professional development, which includes assessment of learning needs, planned learning activity and evaluation. The process should improve patient care, enhance professionalism and motivate practitioners.

Introduction

It goes without saying that general practice in the NHS has grown up during a period of rapid medical and technological advance. During this time general practitioners have endeavoured to maintain their gate-keeping role, as well as developing new skills and expertise to deliver increasingly specialised care in a community setting. The success of chronic disease management programmes and drug-monitoring programmes attests to this capacity for change in general practice.

Over the lifetime of the NHS, concepts of education, learning and development have also evolved. These have enhanced our understanding of individuals, groups and organisations to the point where theory has started to inform both practice and regulation. The theory of adult learning, the idea of the learning cycle, increased sophistication in assessing learning needs, and evaluation of learning have all had an impact in primary care. General practitioners are much more overtly conscious and reflective learners than they were 50 years ago. At the inception of the NHS in 1948, there was still serious debate as to whether general practitioners required any continuing education at all! It was assumed that the knowledge and skills gained at medical school would suffice for a professional lifetime. Today, the proposition is accepted that learning is lifelong and for everyone.

The organisational structure of general practice has also undergone radical change. In the early years of the NHS, general practitioners worked – often single-handed and with minimal receptionist support – from premises which were poorly equipped and lacking essential facilities.[2] There was no concept of a healthcare team, and it was not until the 1960s (when general practitioners were given financial assistance) that improvements in premises, the employment of ancillary staff and the increased size of partnerships led practices to take on the form of 'organisations'. In addition, the greater integration of district nurses, health visitors and midwives in the functioning of the practice meant that even small practices took on an organisational form. The introduction of GP fundholding in 1991 further promoted the concept of an organisational unit, and the basis of the primary healthcare contract in the future may well change from individual general practitioner to primary care organisation. Learning and personal development in the context of an organisation bring their own challenges and opportunities, for general practitioners may have at least two roles, namely boardroom director of the primary care organisation and teamworker on the 'shop-floor'.

What is continuing professional development for?

It is for patient care

Ultimately all professional development activity should benefit patients directly or indirectly. If continuing professional development (CPD) leads to modifications in practice according to research evidence, motivates doctors to view their work positively, leads to better communication with patients, leads to easier or more rapid access to appropriate healthcare and leads to greater public confidence in their doctors, then patients must benefit.

At the individual level, the purpose of much CPD is to produce changes in behaviour. One of the aims of educational research is to discover the best ways of facilitating behavioural change. In contrast, the role of medical and social research is to identify which behaviours or practices lead to health enhancement. When delivering or participating in CPD there is a need to understand what behaviour needs to change and how it needs to do so. Learning methods that make the desired change more likely can then be adopted. This is not to oversimplify the process, for the psychology of learning and adopting change is complex and unique in each individual. Adopting, implementing, embedding and persisting in new behaviours is not a simple matter of 'plug and play'. Change is intensely personal because it requires a person to do something different, think something different and feel something different. People cope with change and react to it in a variety of ways. Senge has postulated a continuum of response to change which moves from apathy to commitment[3] (*see* Figure 6.1). There has been a tendency to decry those who are slow to implement and adopt change (including change as a response to learning) as 'resistors' and 'laggards'. The work of Rogers and Shoemaker[4] and Havelock and colleagues[5] on the diffusion of innovation is often used to support such a contention. However, research focusing on the implementation rather than the adoption of change has shown that there is only limited value in concentrating on the individual as the resistor. The barriers to implementing change are wider than the individual's psychological make-up, and include different values and beliefs, issues of power and control and practical barriers of time, organisation and resources.[6] If CPD is to deliver benefits to patient care, then practitioners undertaking professional development activity, as well as organisers of professional education, need to understand something of both the nature of change and reactions to change.

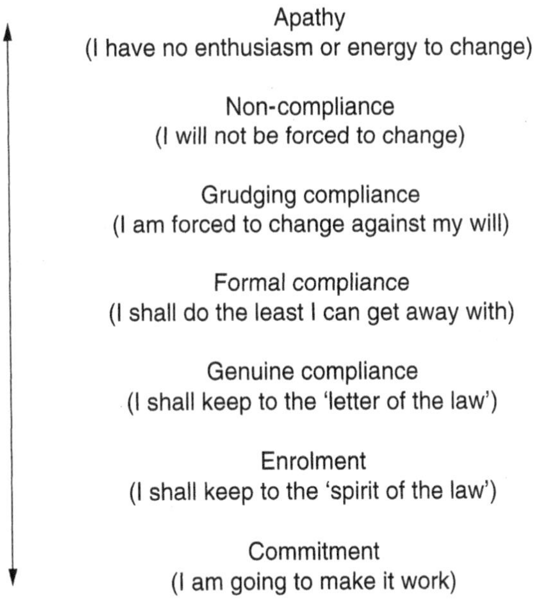

Apathy
(I have no enthusiasm or energy to change)

Non-compliance
(I will not be forced to change)

Grudging compliance
(I am forced to change against my will)

Formal compliance
(I shall do the least I can get away with)

Genuine compliance
(I shall keep to the 'letter of the law')

Enrolment
(I shall keep to the 'spirit of the law')

Commitment
(I am going to make it work)

Figure 6.1   A continuum of response to change (after Senge, 1990).[3]

It is for professionalism

Doctors have two distinct yet overlapping roles – as healer and as professional. The professionalism of doctors relates to how they work within organisational structures in order to deliver the increasingly complex services that are equated with their healer role.[7] Professional status is a privilege that is granted (or revoked) by society, and this makes doctors accountable to society for the trust that society has placed in them. As society becomes more knowledgeable and has more ready access to all kinds of information and, as multiprofessional teamwork develops, doctors are increasingly expected to justify how they understand and apply that discrete body of knowledge and skills which is medicine. Learning and developing as healers and as professionals is no longer a private and personal matter. Professionalism in the twenty-first century demands evidence of learning and development as part of maintaining professional status.

The 'professions' arose out of the guilds and universities of the Middle Ages, and part of being a professional involves taking responsibility for the exercise of one's craft. This operates at a personal level by making sure that one keeps abreast of developments in one's field and that one seeks to practise at a level consistent with such developments. Professionalism also operates at a 'tribal' level, where the professional believes that their behaviour contributes to the reputation of the profession as a whole. It therefore behoves the individual to maintain standards of practice that will not detract from that reputation.

It is for motivation and fulfilment

There are significant extrinsic motivators to encourage general practitioners' participation in CPD. These include money (e.g. the Postgraduate Education Allowance – PGEA), satisfying clinical governance requirements and revalidation. For most doctors these influences play an undisputed role, but there are also intrinsic factors that motivate an individual to participate in CPD.

Maslow postulated a hierarchy of needs which he believed motivated people throughout their lives.[8] A depiction of this hierarchy is presented in Figure 6.2. He postulated that the meeting of one need triggered the motivation to meet the next one above it, and so on. Maslow's hierarchy helps us to understand how motivation to learn can be affected by other unrelated needs in an individual. Continuing professional development produces its beneficial effects by meeting 'growth needs – knowledge needs' (the need to know and understand and to learn about the world around us), 'aesthetic needs' (the need to appreciate the order and balance of life, and to enjoy beauty in the world) and 'self-actualisation needs' (the need to fulfil one's potential in life). 'Growth needs' only become motivators when 'deficiency needs' have been met. Unlike the 'deficiency needs', which cease to motivate once they are satisfied, 'growth needs' continue and grow stronger as they are met. A doctor's under-performance or failure to engage in CPD may reflect unmet 'deficiency needs' such as self-esteem or belonging needs (caused by professional isolation). Until these are addressed, improvement may be difficult.

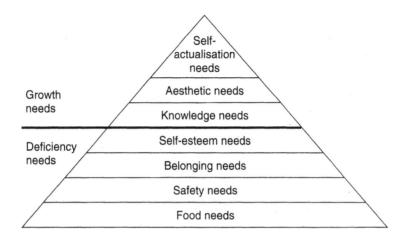

Figure 6.2   Maslow's hierarchy of needs.

Continuing professional development – holistic education

The modern approach to CPD makes explicit what was previously assumed to be implicit. Educational theory and research over the last three decades have generated a number of beliefs (a mixture of research evidence and theoretical postulation) which underpin the modern approach to CPD. These are listed in Box 6.1. This new approach to CPD values more than mere attendance at an organised learning event (as was the case with the requirements for the PGEA introduced in 1990). The new CPD consists of a process which goes beyond simple participation in a learning activity. A useful analogy from the general practice consultation is a doctor advising a patient to stop smoking. Unless the patient recognises a personal need to stop the habit, the advice alone is unlikely to produce change. Similarly, additional activities such as reading a leaflet, attending a support group, using nicotine replacement therapy or having a support-line phone number to ring can all make the change more likely to occur. A follow-up appointment to review the patient and hear what progress has been made towards stopping is also likely to encourage a change in behaviour.

Box 6.1:   Beliefs drawn from educational research and theory of adult learning which underpin the new approach to CPD

- Adults learn throughout their lives.
- The need to know is a powerful motivator for learning.
- Adults are competent to choose what and how to learn.
- Learning is more effective when it is undertaken for a stated reason.
- Learning is more effective when a method is identified and completed.
- Adults prefer learning activities which are problem centred and relevant to their life situation.
- Experience is a rich learning resource, but exposure alone does not guarantee learning.
- Adults wish to apply new learning to their immediate circumstances.
- Learning is more effective when there is some form of follow-up after the learning activity.

The core of CPD is an APPLE

In defining a modern approach to CPD, it is helpful to think in terms of stages in a process. However, it is important to stress that it is a *single* process. The suggested stages are as follows:

- **A**ssessing and identifying needs
- **P**rioritising needs
- **P**lanning learning activity
- **L**earning activity participation
- **E**valuation or follow-up of learning activity.

The following case studies illustrate these stages at work.

Case study 6.1:   Dr George and headache

General practitioner Dr George has recently noticed that a number of patients have presented to her with headaches. She has been uncertain about their diagnosis, but her knowledge of the patients has led her to conclude that tension was the likely cause for most of them. *(At this stage she has **assessed/identified a learning need** in a broad sense.)*

She decides that, in order to feel more certain of her diagnoses, she needs to feel confident about her assessment of patients with headache and the indications for specialist investigation. *(She has now **prioritised her learning need** more specifically.)*

She visits the *British Medical Journal* website and prints off a Fortnightly Review from 1996 which looks helpful. She also speaks to a GP trainer colleague who is able to lend her a video on examining patients with headache. She asks her practice secretary to identify the records of all patients referred by her for a neurological opinion about headache in the last 12 months. Finally, she decides that at some stage she will ring her local neurologist to discuss indications for referral of patients with headache. *(She has now **planned what she intends to do** and located the relevant resources.)*

Dr George wonders how she will know whether her efforts in reading, watching and talking to others will have been worthwhile. She decides that she will be able to recognise her own feeling of increased confidence. She also decides that writing down a personal guideline to use with patients presenting with headache will give her some concrete outcome of her learning, to which she could refer in the future. She also hopes that, by learning more about headache, she might increase the proportion of neurology referrals she makes which are investigated rather than being sent back with no investigations. She realises that any such change might take a year or more to show up. *(Dr George is here considering how she might **evaluate or follow up her learning,** even before she has engaged in any specific learning activity.)*

Over the next couple of weeks, Dr George reads the review article and makes some useful notes. She watches the video and rehearses the examination several times to herself. She also examines the outcomes from her headache referrals over the past year and discovers that only two out of the 10 patients she referred were investigated further. By the time she has done these things, she is pretty sure that she knows when to refer patients for investigation, and her telephone call to the neurologist just confirms what she already knows. She constructs her personal guideline relatively easily, and is gratified to find that she is able to use it twice in the following week, although she discovers it takes more than the average consultation time. She decides that, until she is more competent, she will ask such patients to book a double appointment to allow more time. Three months later she is sufficiently skilled to conduct the assessment within a normal consultation. She also has a feeling that headache patients do not seem to be coming back again and again as much as they were before. Perhaps her diagnostic confidence is making her reassurance more credible.

Twelve months later, she repeats her referral audit and notices that her overall number of headache referrals is down, with more of them being investigated at hospital. In her reflections about what she has learned and experienced, she wonders whether it would be appropriate for the practice nurse to review patients with migraine to ensure that they are being managed correctly. She resolves to raise this issue at a practice meeting. *(Dr George has **completed the CPD process** as far as it related to her initial learning need. But notice how she is beginning to identify a practice and nurse development need. Learning and development are more akin to a spiral than to a cycle.)*

The neat and tidy stages of CPD do not, at first glance, sit well with the day-to-day busyness of patient care and the competing demands on a doctor's time. Sometimes just getting through the day is a worthy achievement! Ideas about CPD can seem unrealistic. The following case study shows how the CPD process can be recognised in a more complex but realistic situation.

Case study 6.2:   On the run with Dr Singh

Going through the practice mail before morning surgery, Dr Singh comes across an executive summary of the latest *National Service Framework on Coronary Heart Disease*, sent on to him by the clinical governance lead of his primary care group (PCG). He does not have time to read it, but notices a few lines about risk scores and cholesterol of 5 mmol/L. He sets it aside, promising himself that he will do something about it later. He also notices that a number of the *random blood sugars* he had requested recently have come back with an asterisk, suggesting an abnormal level, yet as far as he was aware the results were not in the diabetic diagnostic range at all. One of these patients is due to see him that morning, so he takes the result along to his consulting-room as he sets off to start his surgery. His first patient complains: '*I've waited two weeks for this appointment. You must be very popular, Doctor!*' He mutters something about there being a lot of flu about, but reflects that this is not the first time this has been said to him. Such comments also upset him as he prides himself on his punctuality and accessibility. However, he ploughs on. Before the patient with the asterisked random blood sugar result comes in, he rings the laboratory for an explanation about these quasi-abnormal results and discovers, to his slight embarrassment, that the diagnostic criteria for diabetes mellitus have changed! The laboratory agrees to fax him the latest criteria immediately. By the end of morning surgery he is able to look at all those random blood sugar results in the light of the criteria and make a confident assessment. He keeps the fax on his pin-board to refer to in the future. He also wonders what else has changed in diabetes without him knowing! Checking through his repeat prescriptions after surgery is fairly straightforward, although he had to look up a couple of *new drugs*, which patients had been prescribed on discharge from hospital. Before setting off on his two home visits he spends five minutes with his senior receptionist discussing the waiting-times for his appointments. They agree to meet together with the practice manager the following week to see what can be done about it.

In this account, Dr Singh encounters four areas of learning or development need in one morning. He has recognised his need to know, but has sensibly (and intuitively) prioritised them. So the National Service Framework can wait until he has a little more time. If he forgets, it is likely that the PCG will come back to him about it anyway. The issue of the random blood sugars is more immediate, and he completes the CPD process in the course of the morning by identifying the laboratory as his learning resource, speaking to them, obtaining hard copy of the criteria, applying the criteria to his need and keeping the information on hand for continued use. In fact he even begins to recognise that he has a wider learning need in diabetes. He also realises that the problem of appointments requires investigation. He initiates this, involving other team members who will also help him to maintain his motivation to do something about the problem.

Personal development plans (PDPs)

The purpose of this new approach to CPD was examined earlier in the chapter.

- It is a means of improving patient care by changing clinical and organisational practice.
- It is a way of expressing the doctor's accountability to society by providing evidence of continued learning and development.
- It is about attending to the doctor's *growth needs*.

For all these reasons it is important that CPD is recorded in some way. Keeping a record of the process enables the doctor to satisfy those who wish to know that he or she is engaged in learning and development. It also provides the doctor with positive feedback, which motivates further learning and is also testament to continuous quality improvement in patient care.

Documenting their CPD will be a major challenge for many doctors. It does require dedicated time for thinking and writing, as well as a degree of organisation. For the purposes of accountability, doctors need to provide evidence in their documentation of the stages of CPD (APPLE) as it relates to the particular activity being described. The record of CPD is referred to as a personal development plan (PDP), and each doctor will be required to produce one on an annual basis. The PDP is both a prospective plan of intended learning and development, and a record of more opportunistic learning. When planning their intended learning, doctors are expected to identify their learning needs by considering their clinical practice and their practice organisation, as well as local and national priorities. Whether the PDP deals with planned or opportunistic learning, the record needs to reflect the APPLE process where possible. Dr George's record of her learning is shown as an example in Box 6.2.

Box 6.2:   An example of a PDP record

Learning need	Diagnosis and investigation of patients with headache
How was the need identified?	Lack of confidence in dealing with patients with headache Possible over-referral of patients for investigation
Learning activities	Studied review article on headache Watched video on examination of patients with headache Spoke with consultant neurologist
Follow-up of learning	Feel more confident and patients seem more reassured Written personal guideline I examine all new headache patients in the way I learned Decrease in the number of neurology referrals 12 months later

---

Portfolios and folders

It is likely that Dr George's record of learning will contain more than the summary that is reproduced in Box 6.2. It might also include an annotated copy of the review article, notes taken down from reading, her referral audit figures, her personal guideline, and even a copy of the video or notes taken during her telephone conversation with the consultant. She might include her initial thoughts about a nurse-run migraine clinic. All of this 'evidence' comprises her learning portfolio. Some doctors use these portfolios to support their learning further by meeting with colleagues (e.g. their mentors) to reflect on their learning needs and personal development.

Doctors will be required to maintain a folder (portfolio) containing documentary evidence of their CPD for the purposes of revalidation (*see* Chapter 8).

Summary points

- Change in medical practice and organisational structures is unceasing.
- General practitioners have a range of roles in increasingly large primary care organisations, and need to be able to change behaviours accordingly.
- The purpose of much CPD is to achieve behaviour change.
- Complex factors govern an individual's motivation to change, and these need to be understood.
- The process of CPD involves assessing learning needs, planning learning activity and evaluation.
- CPD helps doctors to grow, and can be motivating in itself.
- All doctors will need to document their CPD in a folder for the purposes of revalidation.

References

1   Secretary of State for Health (1998) *A First-Class Service: Quality in the New NHS*. Department of Health, London.

2   Pereira Gray D (1998) Postgraduate training. In: I Loudon, J Horder and C Webster (eds) *General Practice under the National Health Service 1948–1997*. Clarendon Press, Oxford.

3   Senge P (1990) *The Fifth Discipline: the Art and Practice of the Learning Organisation*. Doubleday, New York.

4   Rogers E and Shoemaker F (1971) *Communication of Innovations: A Cross-Cultural Approach*. Free Press, New York.

5   Havelock RG, Huber JC and Zimmerman S (1969) *Major Works on Change in Education: An Annotated Bibliography.* University of Michigan, Ann Arbor, MI.

6   Dalin P (1978) *Limits to Educational Change.* Studies on Education in Change. Macmillan Press Ltd, London.

7   Cruess SR and Cruess RL (1997) Professionalism must be taught. *BMJ.* **315:** 1674–7.

8   Maslow AH (1954) *Motivation and Personality.* Harper and Row, New York.

CHAPTER SEVEN

Appraisal

Di Jelley

No man can reveal to you aught but that which already lies half asleep in the dawning of your knowledge.

The Prophet, Kahlil Gibran

This chapter reviews a range of mechanisms which may be used to contribute to the personal and professional development of general practitioners.

Introduction

The engagement in effective, continuing professional development (CPD), which must be one of the hallmarks of the new GP, requires above all a commitment to lifelong learning and to thoughtful reflective clinical practice. This is not just because of the need to respond to the demands of public expectations and professional regulation described in other chapters. As importantly, general practitioners will only survive as individuals by attending to the needs of self, as well as by practising and learning within an effective multidisciplinary team. In this chapter some of the mechanisms that can be used both by individual general practitioners and by primary care teams to fulfil the requirements of CPD are described. These mechanisms include the following:

- appraisal
- assessment
- mentoring
- supervision
- personal development planning
- practice development planning.

Appraisal, which has long been valued as a powerful motivator in industry and education, is now being advocated for all doctors on an annual basis. Appraisal and assessment are processes that have much in common, but which are often used for different reasons. Mentoring and supervision are also increasingly being discussed in the context of primary care, and may be used in both the training and continuing support of general practitioners and other health professionals. All of these processes may be used as tools in the identification and monitoring of learning and training needs, which form the basis of both personal and practice development plans.

Appraisal

Definition

Appraisal is a well-established process in industry, commerce, the civil service and education, and has been introduced into different sectors of the health service over the past decade. It is primarily an educational process, based on dialogue and interaction with the appraiser, and focusing on the development and training needs of the individual. The main features of appraisal as defined in a recent report[1] are listed in Box 7.1.

Box 7.1:   Key features of appraisal*

- Appraisal is a process that involves collection of information by the appraisee and others followed by a meeting between the appraisee and at least one appraiser for the purpose of reviewing the subject's performance over a range of areas and development objectives.
- The information collected is focused on areas chosen by the appraisee and appraiser within the broader remit of CPD, or defined by the syllabus of the formal training or education programme for doctors in training grades.
- Management appraisal is carried out for the purposes of the organisation rather than the individual subject. In this context, the appraisee's development is viewed in terms of organisational rather than personal goals, although these should also be negotiated to foster personal development.

*Adapted from Standing Committee on Postgraduate Medical Education (1996) *Appraising Doctors and Dentists in Training.*[1]

Appraisal in industry

Appraisal has been used in the commercial sector for many years, and its effectiveness has been extensively studied. The objectives of appraisal in this context are multiple, and include performance appraisal linked to salary review, and identification of strengths, weaknesses and training needs. Hunt, who has researched extensively in this area, explains why evaluations of commercial appraisal highlight both benefits and significant difficulties.[2] He suggests that the breadth and contradictory nature of some of the objectives of performance review (e.g. feedback on self on the one hand and salary review on the other) make it a very difficult process to conduct successfully. He argues that cultural values (e.g. not telling people about their weaknesses) may also militate against its effectiveness. Honesty between bosses and their subordinates may also be a problem, especially if an organisation is under threat. Hunt suggests that appraisal is most likely to work if there can be honest, helpful and constructive feedback, if objectives are jointly set and not imposed, if performance review is related to future objectives and not past failures, and if confidentiality is maintained. He also suggests that '360 degrees' appraisal in which the views of an individual are obtained from management, peers and subordinates is likely to produce the most comprehensive performance review.

Appraisal in education

Performance appraisal has been compulsory for all teachers since 1991. The implications of this requirement, not only for organisational and training reasons but also in terms of securing teachers' commitment to the process, have been considerable. Appraisal has been introduced into schools using a variety of techniques, including direct observation of classes, the use of video recordings, and review of teaching materials and pupils' test results. It has usually been conducted between senior teachers and their junior colleagues. Evaluation of the effectiveness of appraisal has yielded mixed outcomes, again reflecting a wide range of objectives. These have included identifying the strengths and weaknesses of individual teachers, drawing up development plans and improving the management of schools. Some studies report that teachers felt more positive about appraisal once they had actually taken part in it, perceiving it as a tool for personal development rather than a threat. Other reports suggest that the necessary time and resources to establish well-run appraisal systems have not been available – the resulting process being seen as of little use, and as something which is likely to become submerged in the day-to-day routine of school life.

Appraisal in the health service

Experience of the use of appraisal in industry and education can usefully inform its widespread introduction to the health service. Health service managers, practice managers and senior nurses have been using appraisal (discussions between managers and their subordinates) for some years to clarify performance expectations, review progress, recognise achievements and shortfalls, and produce individual development plans. Edis describes in detail how to set up staff appraisal systems in the health service, and also the skills that the appraiser needs to develop.[3] Except for those in management or hospital-based training posts, doctors have largely avoided appraisal until now, but a recent proposal from the Chief Medical Officer (CMO) has changed this perspective.[4] In the document *Supporting Doctors, Protecting Patients*, the following statement was made:

> *Appraisal is a positive process to give someone feedback on their performance, to chart their continuing progress and to identify development needs. It is a forward-looking process essential for the developmental and educational planning needs of the individual ... We propose that appraisal should be made comprehensive and compulsory for all doctors working in the NHS. It is envisaged that appraisal will form an important component of the systems required by the General Medical Council (GMC) for revalidation.*

Box 7.2 describes the link between appraisal and revalidation as described by the General Medical Council. Exactly how appraisal for general practitioners is going to be implemented is not yet clear. There will certainly be time, resource and training implications, if it is to be implemented as a useful and supportive process. There are few existing systems in place, and it seems likely that the Department of Health will work closely with the British Association of Medical Managers (BAMM), who have recently produced a document entitled *Appraisal in Action*. This provides a clear model for appraisal among hospital doctors, both for trainees and between colleagues of equal status. A primary care version is currently being produced.[5]

Peer appraisal in general practice

Definition

Peer appraisal differs from appraisal as discussed in the previous section in one critical way – it takes place between GP colleagues who are usually of equal status, although they may have differing roles and responsibilities within the partnership. The non-hierarchical nature of peer appraisal in general practice may alter both what is being appraised and how the process is conducted. However, some of the same principles apply. Peer appraisal can be described as a process in which GPs meet regularly in pairs or groups to discuss and review their performance and activity in the practice, covering a range of topics. Records are usually kept and a plan is often drawn up focusing on the training and development needs of the GP, linked into practice and local priorities.

Content and process of peer appraisal

There is little published information on peer appraisal in the UK general practice literature, probably because few practices have engaged in it so far. Westcott has described a peer appraisal initiative in Devon,[7] but most of the information in this chapter

---

Box 7.2: Appraisal and the link with revalidation*

- The purpose of appraisal is formative – to support doctors in maintaining and improving their professional performance.
- The appraisal process should include another registered medical practitioner who is professionally accountable to the GMC, in addition to any contractual accountability.
- Appraisal should include (but need not be confined to) a review of a doctor's revalidation folder. Gaps in the information should be identified and filled before the end of the revalidation cycle, so that the assessment is as straightforward as possible.
- Appraisal should identify likely difficulties with a doctor's practice which need to be addressed in the course of the run-up to the assessment at the end of the revalidation cycle. At the end of the cycle there should be no surprises.
- In identifying any difficulties, the appraisal should highlight where these are caused or exacerbated by practice conditions, equipment or levels of staffing.
- Appraisal should ensure that the description of what the doctor does is accurate, and that the information about their fitness to practise is sufficient.
- The appraiser should be able to arrange any developmental or remedial action that is deemed necessary as a result of the appraisal.
- The details of the appraisal discussion should be confidential.
- One outcome of each annual appraisal should be a statement, which will be placed in the revalidation folder, confirming that a satisfactory appraisal process has taken place, and identifying any developmental needs. The agreed statement should be signed and dated by the doctor and the appraiser.
- In exceptional cases where the review of information reveals danger to patients which cannot be resolved by an agreed plan of action, the appraiser must explain to the doctor that, in accordance with every doctor's professional obligation to protect patients, they will be taking whatever steps are necessary to safeguard patients. These might include the types of remedial measures proposed in *Supporting Doctors, Protecting Patients*.

*Adapted from General Medical Council (2000) *Revalidating Doctors. Ensuring Standards, Securing the Future*.[6]

---

comes from a study of peer appraisal I conducted in the Northern Deanery in 1998. All 550 practices were sent a questionnaire and the 24 practices that were identified as having set up peer appraisal systems were interviewed.[8]

As the responsibilities of general practitioners and primary care teams cover such an immense field, peer appraisal can only logistically cover small areas during any appraisal session. The Northern Deanery study suggested that practices approached the content of peer appraisal in a variety of ways, which could be broadly categorised as follows:

- the doctor as an individual and as a team member
- the doctor's educational needs
- the doctor's clinical competence.

In all of the practices, preparation for appraisal required the GP to review their performance (i.e. their strengths and weaknesses) by completing a pre-appraisal pro forma. In some practices this required the collection of data on educational needs by compiling a log diary or by undertaking a computer-based multiple-choice-question programme. Other practices used videos of consultations, records' analysis, Prescribing Analysis and Cost (PACT) data or review of referrals to provide information on clinical performance. In some cases the practice manager also sought feedback on the doctor from members of the administrative and nursing staff. In a system of '360 degrees' appraisal, used in some practices, unidisciplinary groups within a primary care team drew up feedback questionnaires which were then given out to a range of members of the primary care team chosen by the appraisee.

The next stage of the process in all systems of peer appraisal was the appraisal meeting, which might take place between two GP colleagues or a larger group of practice partners, often with the practice manager involved in a facilitatory capacity. A clear structure, protected time and good timekeeping were essential requirements. The meeting started with the appraisee feeding back his or her own views on all aspects of performance chosen for review. The appraiser or other GP colleagues in a group meeting then gave their feedback to the appraisee. The outcome of this process usually highlighted two or three areas where development would benefit both the individual and the practice. These were written up in the appraisal report and formed the basis of that individual's personal development plan. The appraisee specified how these developmental needs would be met, and within what time frame. In '360 degrees' appraisal, feedback from team members was collated by one individual who fed back to each appraisee individually.

Benefits and difficulties of peer appraisal

There is no published systematic evaluation of peer appraisal in the UK. Evidence from industry and education suggests that it is critical that the purpose of appraisal in each specific context is clear. The environment should encourage support and constructive criticism, so that reflective challenge can be accepted by those involved. A recent paper by Peiperl describes a model for evaluating the success of peer review.[9] Her research suggests that feedback from peers is highly valued, especially if the system is well designed and the areas reviewed are directly relevant to the individual's work. Team cohesiveness can be improved through the process of peer review, but the social system in the group must be able to cope with the potential threat of negative feedback.

In the Northern Deanery, two-thirds of the practices interviewed had a positive overall view of peer appraisal. Most of those that did not do so attributed this to partnership factors or to a lack of useful information on how to set up an effective system. Box 7.3 summarises some of the views on appraisal given by the study participants. An important issue relating to appraisal in all situations is the training required by appraisers to give constructive feedback and provide challenge. This has been addressed in a recent article by Haman and Irvine.[10]

Box 7.3:   Benefits and difficulties of peer appraisal

Benefits
1   Improves team cohesion, mutual support and honesty between team members
2   Positive feedback promotes well-being and enthusiasm within the team
3   Facilitates personal and professional development
4   Stimulates thought, reflection and further reading
5   Allows discussion of difficult topics in a 'safe' environment
'Very helpful – every practice should do it'
'Concentrates the mind to think about critical issues'
'Extremely helpful and stimulates me to read'

Difficulties
1   May be difficult to set clear achievable objectives
2   Potential conflict between personal and practice needs
3   Giving negative feedback is difficult, especially in clinical areas
4   Requires time, mutual trust and respect
5   May become safe and non-challenging
'Outcomes of appraisal may be unpredictable ... Some doctors may find it very threatening'

Assessment

Definition

Assessment may involve methods that are also used in appraisal, but its focus is more specific and usually designed to inform the regulatory aspect of career progress. This is the case, for example, in *summative assessment* – an end-point evaluation of GP vocational training, which (typically of assessment) measures performance against external criteria. Unlike appraisal, which aims for consensus between the appraiser and the appraisee, there is no expectation of consensus between the assessor and the assessed. Instead, unbiased and standardised outcomes, based on validity and reliability, are produced by assessment. The main features of assessment[1] are listed in Box 7.4.

Box 7.4:   Main features of assessment*

1   Assessment involves measuring performance in pre-specified tasks, comparing the sub-ject's performance with a fixed standard. These tasks may be real-life service tasks or tests/examinations administered as part of service commitments.
2   Standards may be:
  •   the performance of other people (peer or norm referenced)
  •   a pre-specified set of criteria (criterion referenced)
  •   the assessor's expert understanding of minimum safety requirements.
3   Assessment covers a wide curriculum based on knowledge, clinical skills, attitudes, interpersonal relationships and personal qualities such as leadership potential.

*Adapted from Standing Committee on Postgraduate Medical Education (1996) *Appraising Doctors and Dentists in Training.*[1]

Assessment of clinical competence

Recent highly publicised events, including the Bristol case and the Shipman enquiry, have led to a wholly understandable public and government demand for doctors to demonstrate their clinical competence and to update their clinical skills regularly throughout their professional careers. A more detailed discussion of the proposals for revalidation can be found in Chapter 8. In this section, assessment of clinical competence is discussed only in terms of its relationship to appraisal, and the implications of this for general practitioners in the future.

Southgate has identified a list of competencies,[11] which are summarised in Box 7.5. She argues that two important issues should be taken into account when devising assessments, namely their purpose and content. Is the assessment diagnostic (*formative*) or for licensing purposes (*summative*)? Formative assessment has much in common with appraisal. It identifies learning needs and provides learning opportunities. Summative assessment, on the other hand, drives learning, and it is therefore important to define exactly what will be tested. In this context Southgate suggests the following framework:

1   the problems which the learner will need to solve at the end of training should be identified
2   for each problem, the clinical tasks should be clearly specified
3   a blueprint to guide the selection of problems for the final assessment should be prepared
4   appropriate assessment methods should then be chosen.

Both competence (what the doctor is capable of doing) and performance (what the doctor actually does) form part of assessment. The literature on both is vast and is beyond the scope of this chapter. The importance of assessment in this context is to learn from experience in the fields of education and management, and thereby to inform the introduction of appraisal in the context of general practice. Criteria and methods which are chosen as part of the appraisal process must be seen to reflect the complex reality of general practice. Doctors need to believe that reviewing and assessing their performance is a valid, reliable process that contributes not only to their personal development, but also to improved service provision.

Box 7.5:   Tasks of a competent clinician*

The main tasks are as follows:

- to deliver curative and rehabilitative care
- to promote health and organise preventative activity
- to plan and evaluate health education activities
- to collaborate with agents of community development
- to participate in research and teaching
- to manage services and resources
- to learn with/train other members of the health team
- to engage in self-directed learning and self-evaluation.

*Adapted from Southgate (1994).[11]

Supervision

Definition

Supervision is a term most often associated with the education, training and support of professionals in the fields of social work, counselling, psychology and psychotherapy. It has been defined in a self-development manual by Knapman and Morrison as:

> *A process in which one worker is given responsibility to work with another worker in order to achieve certain professional, personal and organisational objectives. These objectives include competent, accountable practice, continuing professional development and personal support.*[12]

They argue that supervision is a vital tool for identifying knowledge, concerns, observations, ideas, role and contribution, and as such is a key vehicle for professional development.[12] The purposes of supervision as described in their manual are listed in Box 7.6. Fish and Twinn maintain that it is the educational aspect of supervision that determines its quality. They have reviewed the role of supervision in a range of health professions, and conclude that as pressure to demonstrate sustained high-quality practice increases, so does the need for educational supervision, both during and after completion of professional training. They further suggest that the role of the supervisor is not just to facilitate learning and assess competence, but also to encourage practitioners to reflect and so develop their professional expertise.[13] Supervision has other functions in addition to being educational. It can play a managerial role, providing an overview of a trainee's performance and thus incorporating some elements of quality control that are more allied to summative assessment than to appraisal. Supervision should also be supportive, providing a trusting relationship in which the supervisor can identify the personal impact of their intervention. In addition, it can play a mediating role, establishing feedback mechanisms between the organisation and the individual, and vice versa.

Box 7.6:   The purposes of supervision*

These include the following:

- maintaining and developing the quality of practice
- professional development – the opportunity to learn, explore and deepen understanding of practice
- role clarity – to define role boundaries and expectations
- organisation objectives – clarification of the role of the individual in relation to the needs of the organisation
- promoting a suitable climate for practice
- stress reduction
- communication – to provide a mechanism for effective two-way communication
- resources – to discuss the resources needed for the job.

*Adapted from Knapman and Morrison (1999).[12]

Perhaps one of the most important aspects of supervision with regard to appraisal is the overlap of skills required by the competent supervisor or appraiser. One of the most critical skills in either context is that of giving constructive feedback. Some basic rules for giving feedback from Russell's book, *Effective Feedback Skills*,[14] are listed in Box 7.7. There is evidence that these skills can be developed and improved with appropriate training.[14] The practice of supervision has not yet been incorporated into general practice, although some educators argue that much of GP registrar in-practice training is a form of clinical supervision.[15] Given the evidence that well-structured supervision can both improve the quality of care provided and relieve stress on individual practitioners, and given the clear links between supervision and appraisal, it seems likely that supervision will play an increasing role in CPD for general practitioners, perhaps most importantly for single-handed practitioners who lack an easily accessible peer group.

Box 7.7:   Rules for giving feedback

1   It should be balanced.
2   It should be specific.
3   It should be objective.
4   It should be appropriate.
5   It should be understandable.
6   It should be participative.
7   It should be comparable.
8   It should be actionable.

Mentoring

Definition

Mentoring is another process which is likely to play an increasingly important role in general practitioners' CPD. Mentoring has been described in a recent Standing Committee on Postgraduate Medical Education (SCOPME) report as:

> *The process whereby an experienced, highly regarded, empathic person (the mentor) guides the mentee in the development and re-examination of their own ideas, learning and personal and professional development.*[16]

Mentoring and supervision overlap in their aims and roles in professional training and development, but they are not co-terminous. Supervisors usually have a more formal responsibility for delivery of a product (e.g. safe and competent social worker or counsellor). The well-being and personal development of the supervisee represent only one part of the process, in contrast to mentoring, where the development of the mentee is the primary focus. Mentoring has been described as a broad approach to encourage human growth, particularly if the mentor can provide – through their own insight or wisdom – exceptional learning experiences for the mentee.

A number of different models have been proposed as a framework for delivering mentoring, and they are all underpinned by the concept of reflective practice. The work of Egan is one example of a cycle in which current practice is explored and reviewed, the preferred vision is discussed, and action strategies to achieve changes are put into place, before the new reality is again reviewed.[17]

Mentoring is currently taking place in general practice, and several accounts of mentoring schemes for newly qualified or established GPs have been published.[18,19] Freeman, in her textbook on mentoring,[20] suggests that the development of mentoring in general practice owes its origins to the crisis of organisational change. She argues that the recent pace of change in general practice has led to the use of mentors to reduce the isolation and anxiety caused by change. She suggests that mentoring in general practice has three main roles:

- personal support
- continuing education
- professional development

and that it is a particularly useful mechanism during stages of transition (e.g. the shift from GP registrar to new principal, the return from a career break, or a change in career focus).[20]

Competent mentoring requires similar skills to those found in appraisal, formative assessment and supervision. These include the skills of coaching, giving feedback and encouragement, promoting networking, facilitation, counselling, providing supportive challenge and acting as a role model. If delivered appropriately, mentoring has the potential to contribute significantly to the appraisal process, particularly in the area of personal development and management of self.

Personal and practice development planning

Definition

Continuing professional development has been defined as a process of lifelong learning which enables individuals to fulfil their potential while at the same time meeting the requirements of patients and the NHS (*see* Chapter 6). Doctors can only continue to develop professionally by engaging in a continuing reflective and challenging educational process. Personal and practice development planning is now advocated as a key mechanism whereby general practitioners can engage in professional education and personal development.

Personal development plans

Logically, the production of a personal development plan follows on from any of the activities described in this chapter. The key element in all of these processes is engagement in reflective practice – repeatedly asking the following questions.

- What am I doing now?
- How well am I doing it?
- Could I do it better?
- How could I improve my performance?
- Am I doing better now?

Appraisal provides a clear structure for responding to these questions in the context of individual or group interviews. Assessment, supervision and mentoring can also contribute to the processes of identifying educational needs and reviewing performance.

A range of tools is available for defining learning needs.[21] Once the individual doctor has identified a list of their personal needs, interests and aspirations, these can then be discussed within the partnership in order to prioritise personal needs alongside practice needs and so produce both an individual personal development plan and a practice plan. The personal plan will generally result from an annual appraisal meeting. Its detailed structure will vary between practices, but it is likely to contain a list of objectives, methods by which they will be achieved, outcome measures and a defined time frame in which to meet them. Personal development plans will form part of the documentary evidence that is needed for revalidation, and doctors will need to keep them in their folders.

Practice development plans

The practice development plan sets out the practice's strategic direction for education and development. Jones suggests that practice development plans combine documented personal learning needs with practice needs, and also take into account local and national NHS priorities.[22] The practice plan should include all doctors within the practice (including retainers and long-term locums), and can be extended to include other members of the primary care team. The plan must indicate how the success of planned activities can be assessed (e.g. through clinical audit or the implementation of guidelines).

The ultimate aims of the practice development plan will be to set objectives and priorities for future years, to provide an important link with the primary care group or trust, and to demonstrate the practice's achievements with regard to local and national priorities. Regular staff and partner appraisal, promoting a culture of reflective practice, will play an important role in the formulation of this important document.

Conclusion

The CPD of general practitioners is moving away from attendance at accredited educational events towards personal development plans, and this shift requires the development of supportive mechanisms. Activities such as appraisal and mentoring should help doctors not only to survive the rigours of revalidation, but also to thrive in the new NHS.

Sources of information

Guidance on setting up peer appraisal in general practice, which could be applied not only to doctors but also to other members of the primary care team, can be found in the following sources.

A Peer Appraisal Package – some ideas for GPs who want to set up a peer appraisal system in their practice

This is written by Dr Di Jelley and may be obtained from Beverley Brennan, Postgraduate Institute of Medicine and Dentistry, University of Newcastle, 10–12 Framlington Place, Newcastle upon Tyne NE2 4AB, UK (tel 0191 222 6766).

The Good CPD Guide – A Practical Guide to Managed CPD

This is edited by Janet Grant, Ellie Chambers and Gordon Jackson, and may be obtained from Reed Healthcare Publishing, Quadrant House, Sutton, Surrey SM2 5AS, UK (tel 020 8652 8789).

Clinical Insight

A computer-based program used to support a '360 degrees' appraisal model in primary care. It is available from Edgecumbe Health Ltd, Edgecumbe Hill, Clifton, Bristol BS8 1AT, UK (tel 0117 973 8899).

Further reading

Rughani A (2000) *The GP's Guide to Personal Development Plans*. Radcliffe Medical Press, Oxford.
While R and Attwood M (eds) (2000) *A Practitioner's Guide to Professional Development*. Blackwell Science, Oxford.

Summary points

- Engagement in effective CPD will be one of the hallmarks of the new GP.
- There is a range of mechanisms in use in the commercial sector, education and the health service, which promote the necessary reflection on practice.
- Most of these require discussion – between the subject and their appraiser, mentor or supervisor.
- Annual appraisal of general practitioners will support their CPD *and* contribute to their revalidation. Appraisal and revalidation are linked.
- Personal development plans can be produced from appraisal, and will form part of the documentary evidence that is needed for revalidation.
- There is relatively little experience of appraisal or of the other mechanisms in general practice, but peer appraisal is thought to be beneficial.
- In contrast to the other mechanisms, assessment is based on comparison with external criteria and standards.

References

1 Standing Committee on Postgraduate Medical and Dental Education (1996) *Appraising Doctors and Dentists in Training.* Standing Committee on Postgraduate Medical and Dental Education, London.

2 Hunt J (1992) *Managing People at Work* (3e). McGraw Hill International, Maidenhead.

3 Edis M (1995) *Performance Management and Appraisal in the Health Services.* Kogan Page, London.

4 Chief Medical Officer (1999) *Supporting Doctors, Protecting Patients.* NHS Executive, Department of Health, London.

5 British Association of Medical Managers (1999) *Appraisal in Action.* British Association of Medical Managers, Stockport.

6 General Medical Council (2000) *Revalidating Doctors. Ensuring Standards, Securing the Future.* General Medical Council, London.

7 Westcott R (1998) Who's for appraisal? *Educ Gen Pract.* **9**: 447–51.

8 Jelley D and van Zwanenberg T (2000) Peer appraisal in general practice: a descriptive study in the Northern Deanery. *Educ Gen Pract.* **11**: 281–7.

9 Pieperl M (1999) Conditions for the success of peer evaluation. *Int J Hum Resource Manag.* **10**: 429–58.

10 Haman H and Irvine S (1998) Appraisal for general practice development. *Educ Gen Pract.* **9**: 44–50.

11   Southgate L (1994) Freedom and discipline: clinical practice and the assessment of clinical competence. *Br J Gen Pract*. **44**: 87–92.

12   Knapman J and Morrison T (1999) *Making the Most of Supervision in Health and Social Care*. Pavilion Publishing, Brighton.

13   Fish D and Twinn S (1997) *Quality Clinical Supervision in the Health Care Professions*. Butterworth-Heinemann, London.

14   Russell TG (1994) *Effective Feedback Skills*. Kogan Page, London.

15   Rutt G (1994) Vocational training – teaching or supervision? *Educ Gen Pract*. **5**: 274–7.

16   Standing Committee on Postgraduate Medical Education (1998) *An Enquiry into Mentoring – Supporting Doctors and Dentists at Work*. Standing Committee on Postgraduate Medical Education, London.

17   Egan G (1998) *The Skilled Helper* (6e). Brooks/Cole, USA.

18   Alliot R (1996) Facilitating mentoring in general practice. *BMJ*. Classified Suppl. 28 Sept.

19   Bregazzi R, Harrison J and van Zwanenberg T (2000) Mentoring new GPs: experience from GP career start in County Durham. *Educ Gen Pract*. **11**: 58–64.

20   Freeman R (1999) *Mentoring in General Practice*. Butterworth-Heinemann, London.

21   Eve R (2000) Learning with PUNS and DENS. *Educ Gen Pract*. **11**: 73–7.

22   Jones-Elwyn G (1998) Professional and practice development plans for primary care teams. *BMJ*. **316**: 1619–20.

CHAPTER EIGHT

Revalidation for clinical general practice

Mike Pringle

This chapter explores the principles underlying revalidation, and describes how they are being applied in general practice. Revalidation is one of the systems of quality assurance in the health service, and it interacts with the other systems (e.g. clinical governance).

Introduction

The General Medical Council (GMC) has decided that all doctors will, at intervals, demonstrate their continuing fitness to practise.[1] For 36 000 general practitioners this has significant implications.

Background

Prior to the Medical Act of 1858, medicine was a commercial enterprise only regulated by common law. As medicines became more potent and interventions became more aggressive, the GMC was created to protect the public both from charlatans and from exploitation.[2] Until the 1980s, the GMC was primarily concerned with two activities, namely running a register of qualified doctors, and responding to behaviour among those doctors that would either bring the profession into disrepute or exploit patients in the doctor–patient relationship.

It was not until the 1980s that the GMC became concerned about the possibility of ill health in doctors putting patients at risk. Most obviously there was concern about psychological illnesses, especially alcohol and drug abuse, but other illnesses are also covered by the health procedures. These procedures do not usually take the form of a 'trial', but aim to resolve the risk to patients quickly and effectively by other means.

Only in the last decade has the GMC woken up to its responsibilities in the area of performance. Its complex and detailed performance procedures have still only been used on rare occasions, but the cases concerned have revealed an astonishing level of under-performance among some of the doctors concerned.

Finally, in November 1998, the General Medical Council decided to back the idea of revalidation of all doctors at regular intervals – the obligation to demonstrate continuing fitness to practise. The system will not be introduced until May 2001, and it will take up to five years to revalidate all doctors. It is a major bureaucratic and organisational exercise, and it represents a decisive move from reactive regulation (responding when things go wrong) to proactive regulation (detecting under-performance before disaster strikes). It must be asked why it is necessary to go to such lengths.

The answer is that the future of professional regulation demands it. A series of high-profile cases have been interpreted as evidence that the old reactive system of regulation does not work. The Bristol paediatric heart surgery case,[3] the gynaecologists Rodney Ledward and Richard Keale, and then Harold Shipman,[4] the multiple murderer, have heightened anxieties about the risk to which patients are unwittingly exposed.

Despite the fact that revalidation would not, for example, have detected Harold Shipman, the public and political pressure for enhanced regulation seems unstoppable. Moreover, many doctors welcome the opportunity to demonstrate that they are delivering a quality service, and the fact that gross under-performance will at last be dealt with effectively.

The state's concern about poor performance has also become clear. In his report, *Supporting Doctors, Protecting Patients*,[5] the Chief Medical Officer proposed an NHS structure that would enhance the state's role in regulation and reduce the profession's input.

What is revalidation?

Revalidation is the periodic demonstration of fitness to practise. However, that simple sentence skates over a large number of issues. The ground rules are still being refined, and this chapter is based on current understandings in the middle of the year 2000.

Revalidation will not just occur as a 'sudden death' event – a summative assessment – every five years. It will be linked to continuing professional development,[6] regular appraisal and clinical governance.[7] Every doctor will be expected to be on course for a successful revalidation throughout the five years. Where doubts are raised these will be dealt with at the time, and not deferred until the five years have elapsed.

Almost all of the evidence that we expect general practitioners to submit will be collected for other purposes such as clinical governance and continuing professional development. The intention is to ensure that revalidation involves the minimum effort for the maximum efficiency in identifying and addressing under-performance.

How will we know whether it works?

The acid test is the detection of under-performance. The combination of subjective assessment through regular peer appraisal, and objective measures through the evidence submitted, should detect patterns of poor performance but will not necessarily find either isolated (in one very restricted area of practice) under-performance or well-disguised criminality.

All of the evidence from the GMC's performance procedures suggests that poorly performing doctors usually perform badly across a whole range of areas. Revalidation for GPs has therefore been designed to detect such patterns. If cases emerge where patterns of poor performance have not been detected by revalidation, then the system will need to be developed further to make it more robust.

In addition to the reliable detection of serious under-performance, revalidation must be credible in the eyes of the public. If they consider that it is a sham which does nothing to protect them, then it will not matter how good it is in reality. It will not be 'fit for purpose'. Equally, it must command the support of the vast majority of the medical profession. It cannot be imposed upon an unwilling profession.

It must also encourage good practice, and should not create perverse incentives for poor care. It must be equitable to all doctors regardless of gender, age or ethnicity, whether or not they work in the NHS, whether they are part-time or full-time, and whether they are salaried or self-employed.

The final test will be one of efficiency. Revalidation must be realistic and deliverable. It cannot be a nightmare involving reams of paper and hundreds of practice visits, and it cannot cost thousands of pounds and distract clinicians from caring for patients. These are tough criteria for the system of revalidation to meet.

The story so far

The GMC knows that it cannot deliver revalidation on the ground. It is looking to the Royal Colleges and professional associations for the design and management of the system within the GMC's guidelines and to GMC standards. In November 1998, the Royal College of General Practitioners established a Revalidation Working Group on to which it invited representatives of the General Practitioners' Committee of the British Medical Association, patients from the College's Patient Liaison Group, and representatives from the National Association of Non-Principals, the Overseas Doctors Association, the National Association of GP Tutors, the Committee of General Practice Education Directors and the Joint Committee for Postgraduate Training in General Practice. The GMC has observer status and ensures that the group's work is consistent with its plans.

This Revalidation Working Group has published a consultation document entitled *Revalidation for Clinical General Practice*,[8] to which there were nearly 2000 responses. These were overwhelmingly positive, but with major reservations about the workload and potential cost.

The next tasks for the Working Group include specifying the precise criteria, standards and evidence that will be expected from general practitioners, with consultation on these scheduled for late 2000. The group is also attempting to design the detailed organisation of revalidation for general practitioners. The contents of this chapter reflect my understanding of what is likely to emerge from those deliberations, but cannot at this stage be taken as the definitive answer.

What are the standards against which doctors will be assessed?

It is essential that all doctors know what is expected of them and what criteria will be used to assess them. This cannot be a capricious exercise with different standards applied to different individuals, groups or geographical areas.

All doctors will be revalidated against the GMC's document *Good Medical Practice.*[9] The Royal College of General Practitioners convened a group (which included most of the professional groups in the Revalidation Working Group) that has written *Good Medical Practice for General Practitioners.*[10] This was sent out for consultation, and has been supported in a ratio of 15 to 1 by general practitioners.

Good Medical Practice for General Practitioners puts flesh on the bare bones of *Good Medical Practice* in the context of general practice, and then defines the characteristics of an excellent GP and those of an unacceptable GP. It is the latter attributes against which a general practitioner will be assessed for revalidation.

What evidence will be required?

The likely first evidence will be a self-assessment against the attributes of the unacceptable GP in *Good Medical Practice for General Practitioners*, and a signed statement that these do *not* apply. This statement will be supported by signed statements from each regular appraisal to show first that these have occurred, secondly that they have been satisfactory and thirdly that they have not revealed problems that should jeopardise revalidation. For example, if the general practitioner is not taking part in continuing professional development or audits show a very poor level of care, the appraiser will not sign the doctor up, and early assessment will occur.

There will then be a number of areas in which evidence will be required to show that revalidation can be justified (*see* Box 8.1). For general practitioners, the only major area which requires evidence that is not routinely collected for other purposes is communication skills. At present it is envisaged that there will be a number of methodologies approved nationally, and that at least one will involve giving a validated and reliable questionnaire to, say, 50 consecutive consulting patients.

The GP will submit a folder (*see* Box 8.2) incorporating their personal development plan or portfolio that covers their continuing professional educational activity. They will

---

Box 8.1: Information for revalidation*

The information for revalidation will need to be collected and assessed under the following general headings:

1   good clinical care
2   maintaining good medical practice (keeping up to date)
3   relationship with patients
4   working with colleagues
5   teaching and training
6   probity
7   health.

*From General Medical Council (2000) *Revalidating Doctors. Ensuring Standards, Securing the Future.*[11]

Box 8.2: The revalidation folder*

The folder will:

- contain the doctor's relevant personal details
- describe what the doctor does
- contain information to demonstrate the doctor's performance, and describe the steps the doctor is taking to stay up to date and to develop professionally. This information should be collected against each of the headings of *Good Medical Practice* (*see* Box 8.1)
- confirm that the information has been reviewed and an action plan agreed.

Information about performance should come from a wide range of sources including, wherever possible, the doctor, his or her patients, the doctor's colleagues and the doctor's managers.
    Doctors will be expected to provide information on the following:

- their pattern of performance
- continuing professional development (CPD)
- critical incidents (where appropriate)
- patient complaints and compliments
- the results of any external assessments (e.g. Royal College or Deanery accreditation for training).

*From General Medical Council (2000) *Revalidating Doctors. Ensuring Standards, Securing the Future.*[11]

---

also list all formal complaints that they have received, and give an account of how they responded to them. They will state that a minimum range of equipment is available to them, and submit their regular clinical audits. An audit of their medical records will show a legible entry for all consultations of sufficient detail to allow another doctor to take over the patient's care. They will show acceptable access to their services, evidence of teamworking, reasonable referral practice and effective prescribing.

The organisation of revalidation

When a general practitioner's name comes up for revalidation, we expect that the material gathered will be sent to a local revalidation group. There it is proposed that three individuals – a GP local to the doctor, a GP who works some distance away, and a lay person – will look at the material. In the vast majority of cases, the doctor's submission will be supported, the GMC will be notified and the doctor will be revalidated.

If there are doubts, then further information will be sought, probably by a process that includes a practice visit. If problems are identified, then support will be required to help the doctor to put those problems right. Only if a general practitioner will not or cannot improve (or where their continued practice would endanger patients) will the GMC be notified. The local revalidation group can support a doctor's revalidation but it cannot 'de-validate' anyone. That is the business of the GMC's performance procedures. Thus the local group will either recommend revalidation or refer the doctor to the GMC's performance or other (e.g. health) procedures.

A national group will audit the working of the local revalidation groups to ensure that they are discharging their roles responsibly and fairly. In turn, the GMC will need to be satisfied that revalidation is rigorous, consistent and equitable.

Other issues

The description here relates to the revalidation of a clinical general practitioner. All of the criteria and evidence will be tailored to meet the special circumstances of non-principals as well as principals. However, there are complexities with regard to non-core general practice services and non-clinical activities.

Doctors will be asked to describe what they do. Those who say that they work in clinical general practice will be revalidated in a standard system, as described above. In addition, some doctors may say that they offer special clinical care (e.g. colposcopy or drug addiction services), and many will declare that they are involved in management, teaching, research and so on.

For each of these areas the doctor will be asked to show that, as appropriate, they were properly trained for the task, they are keeping their skills up to date, they are regularly appraised in that area and their performance is satisfactory.

Some doctors will take a career break and will not wish to be revalidated when their time is due, but may wish to return later. Others will wish to take on new activities that were not included in their last revalidation. In these circumstances, the doctor will be expected to work in a supervised capacity until he or she is competent, and to send evidence of that competency to the local revalidation group. Thus a returner to general practice, for example, would be supervised by another general practitioner until evidence of reaching the standards required for revalidation had been obtained. This might take a few days or much longer, depending on the extent to which clinical skills have atrophied.

The last and most difficult issue is the extent to which the process results in assessment of the practice as opposed to assessment of the individual doctor. All of the evidence for revalidation will be personal to that doctor, and it is the one doctor who is being revalidated. However, there is the possibility that a halo effect might artificially enhance the performance of a poorly performing doctor who happened to be working in a very good practice. There are no easy answers to this problem, but over time revalidation will need to become sensitive enough to address it.

Conclusion

It seems that revalidation is here to stay. Our prime responsibility now is to design a system that meets the expectations of the public and the profession, offering the maximum protection for the minimum effort. The scheme for revalidation described here is intended to meet those expectations.

Summary points

- All doctors will be required to demonstrate, on a regular basis, their continuing fitness to practise through the process of revalidation.
- The process is intended to be continuous, so that under-performance can be recognised and addressed at an early stage.
- Periodically, doctors will be required to submit a folder to a local revalidation group, which will recommend (or not) revalidation by the GMC.
- If revalidation is not recommended, the doctor in question will be referred to the GMC's performance or other (e.g. health) procedures.
- General practitioners' folders will contain evidence about their performance against the standards set out in *Good Medical Practice for General Practitioners*, and will be derived from a variety of sources.
- Revalidation represents a shift away from reactive regulation (responding when things go wrong) and towards proactive regulation (detecting under-performance before things go wrong).

References

1   General Medical Council (1998) *Press Release.* General Medical Council, London.

2   Tudor Hart J (1988) *A New Kind of Doctor.* Merlin Press, London.

3   Smith R (1998) All changed, changed utterly. *BMJ.* **316**: 1917–18.

4   Pringle M (2000) The Shipman Inquiry: implications for the public's trust in doctors. *Br J Gen Pract.* **50**: 355–6.

5   Department of Health (1999) *Supporting Doctors, Protecting Patients.* Department of Health, London.

6   Chief Medical Officer (1998) *A Review of Continuing Professional Development in General Practice.* Department of Health, London.

7   Royal College of General Practitioners (1999) *Practice Advice on the Implementation of Clinical Governance in England and Wales.* Royal College of General Practitioners, London.

8   The Revalidation Working Group (2000) *Revalidation for Clinical General Practice.* Royal College of General Practitioners, London.

9   General Medical Council (1998) *Good Medical Practice.* General Medical Council, London.

10 Good Medical Practice Working Group (2000) *Good Medical Practice for General Practitioners.* Royal College of General Practitioners, London.

11 General Medical Council (2000) *Revalidating Doctors. Ensuring Standards, Securing the Future.* General Medical Council, London.

CHAPTER NINE

Clinical governance

George Taylor

Clinical governance aims to bring together managerial, organisational and clinical approaches to improving quality of care. If successful, it will define a new kind of professionalism for the next century.

Buetelow and Rowland[1]

This chapter explores the relatively new concept of clinical governance. Although primarily concerned with quality improvement, clinical governance must also tackle poor performance in both individuals and teams.

Introduction

The idea of clinical governance was first introduced into the NHS by the New Labour government in its 1997 White Paper *The New NHS: Modern, Dependable.*[2] It formed part of a series of developments aimed at improving the state and quality of healthcare.[3] Clinical governance was intended to be a '*framework through which NHS organisations are accountable for continuously improving the quality of their services and safeguarding high standards of care by creating an environment in which excellence in clinical care will flourish.*' No one could therefore doubt the new government's commitment to improving standards of clinical care and accountability.

The White Paper identified ten components of clinical governance (*see* Box 9.1).

Responsibility for implementing clinical governance was given to the new primary care groups (PCGs) and primary care trusts (PCTs). Each PCG was required to appoint a clinical governance lead, and each practice within a PCG was required to identify a practitioner responsible for clinical governance. This is perhaps not as revolutionary as it might at first appear for, as the Royal College of General Practitioners (RCGP) has

---

Box 9.1:   The ten commandments of clinical governance[2]

- Quality improvement processes integrated with the quality programme for the organisation
- Leadership skill development at clinical team level
- Evidence-based practice with an infrastructure to support it
- Dissemination of good ideas and innovations
- Clinical risk reduction programmes
- Open investigation of adverse events, and lessons learned promptly applied
- Lessons learned from patients' complaints
- Poor clinical performance identified early and dealt with
- Clinical governance reflected in professional development programmes
- High-quality data to monitor clinical care

---

indicated, clinical governance is '*largely a new name for established concepts: a framework for the improvement of patient care through commitment to high standards, reflective practice, risk management, and personal and team development.*'[4]

The RCGP identified three key concepts within clinical governance, namely protecting patients, developing people and developing teams and systems (*see* Box 9.2).

Box 9.2:   Key concepts of clinical governance[4]

Protecting patients	Identifying unacceptable variations in care
	Managing and minimising poor performance in colleagues
	Risk management
Developing people	Lifelong learning
	Protocols for best practice
	Personal accreditation
	Recognising success
Developing teams and systems	Learning from others
	Audit
	Guideline development
	Celebrating success
	Evidence-based medicine
	Improved cost-effectiveness
	Listening to patients
	Practice accreditation
	Development of accountability and transparency

As a consequence of implementing a clinical governance programme, several outcomes should occur. First, one would expect to see new quality assurance mechanisms. These would cover both individual practitioners and the organisations where they work, protecting both patients individually and the interests of patients as a whole. Secondly, clinical governance should lead to a higher level of professionalism, helping GPs to keep up to date, maintaining and developing standards and, most importantly, protecting the public from malpractice. Thirdly, clinical governance should generate a new culture of lifelong learning, where learning is valued both for the individual's own professional development and also as a means of improving the quality of the wider NHS.

Quality and its measurement

Central to the government's commitment to clinical governance is the attempt to improve the quality of care. We feel that we know instinctively what quality of care is, but attempts to define it show that quality has proved to be a rather flexible concept. Some have defined quality of care narrowly in terms of its impact on patient outcomes,[5] some have linked it to the cost of treatment,[6] while others have focused on the factors needed to achieve quality.[7] One approach to the notion of quality of care which meshes quite well with the framework of clinical governance is a concern for the overall environment of care (*see* Box 9.3).

Box 9.3:   The quality environment[8]

- An appropriate climate for quality
- Serving client interests
- Supporting and developing staff
- Improving policy and practice
- Constant review and evaluation based on valid information

However it is defined, some type of auditing process is needed to measure and assess the quality of care. This process has been called by many names, notably 'clinical audit' when it is multidisciplinary and 'medical audit' when it relates only to doctors. On occasion, the term 'measurement of clinical effectiveness' has been used. Officially, audit has been defined as *'the systematic, cyclical analysis of the quality of medical care, including the procedures used for diagnosis and treatment, the use of resources, and the resulting outcome and quality of life for the patient'.*[9]

To be effective, audit must indeed be a cyclical activity.[10] The cycle consists of four steps (*see* Box 9.4).

Box 9.4:   The audit cycle

• Develop a standard of care.
• Collect data.
• Compare data against the standard.
• Decide whether the standard needs to be modified or whether care needs to be modified.

The audit cycle can be entered at any point, but it must be completed. It is not quite so straightforward to implement as it appears. For example, merely collecting and discussing the data does not constitute a proper audit. Standards may not be set at all, or they may not be set scientifically. Moreover, the review process is a complex activity. Audit decisions may be influenced by a wide range of factors (e.g. peer pressure, the relative education and persuasiveness of different participants, the skill with which a product under test is marketed, or budgetary constraints). Surveys suggest that the proportion of all audits which are conducted with adequate scientific rigour may be as low as 5%.[11]

Three distinct groups are involved in the delivery and audit of quality care, namely clinicians, managers and patients. Each of these groups will have its own particular priorities so far as audit is concerned.[12] If clinical governance is to be completely successful, then quality improvement must involve each of these groups, and their different perspectives, as far as is possible.

Clinicians and quality

A range of methods is available to clinicians to help them to monitor the quality of care they deliver. Some examples are listed below.

Routine performance monitoring

This refers to the keeping and analysing of statistics relating to workload, prescribing, hospital referrals, and so on. Routine statistics will sometimes be collected at the request of the health authority, or else they may be gathered as an internal practice activity. The review and discussion of practice statistics can be one method of internal audit.

Significant event auditing[13]

Here teams carry out an in-depth analysis of a particular incident and the factors that led up to it – either where something has gone wrong, or where there is cause for celebration because something has gone particularly well. Such audits have the value of being multidisciplinary in nature, and they can be used as an internal developmental activity.

Surveys of patients

Questionnaire surveys or interviews with patients can be used to assess levels of satisfaction with the services that the practice provides.

Observation of consultations

Doctors in training for general practice must now record their consultations on videotape, both to facilitate their professional development and as a means of assessing their competence. General practice trainers are also expected to have their teaching and consulting reviewed by colleagues.[14] This is carried out either by direct observation or by viewing videotapes. The direct observation of established GPs' consultations is frequently proposed, but as yet is rarely carried out.

Peer appraisal

Peer appraisal should involve helping the other to improve, rather than merely trying to unearth poor performance. A small number of practices do now conduct mutual appraisal.[15] However, doctors are generally diffident about appraising or assessing their colleagues, the unwritten rule being that one does not question the actions of another professional.[8]

Managers and quality

The establishment in the 1990s of medical audit advisory groups (MAAGs) and GP fundholding brought quality issues into the primary care contracting process, albeit with rather mixed results. MAAGs introduced the idea of audit to those who had limited previous experience of it, and they provided audit tools for many practices. However, they failed to establish convincing methods of quality assessment across the NHS.[1]

GP fundholding allowed primary care to question some of the standards of secondary care. In many ways it opened the door to the development of internal quality systems. Fundholding might have been poorly directed and expensive in terms of outcome, but at least it introduced many practitioners to the concept of audit.[16] With fundholding, hospitals and general practitioners became involved to a greater or lesser degree in the regular audit of their work. Fundholding also provided mechanisms for greater financial control within the NHS, leading to explicit rationing of services in some areas – where only a limited sum of money was available, a finite number of operations could be funded. If a treatment was found to be ineffective, health authorities were less likely to fund it. This limiting of funding was regarded as an improvement in quality by some.[17,18] However, various studies by the Audit Commission indicate that, overall, fundholding failed to bring about significant improvements in quality.[19,20]

The new Labour government of 1997 moved primary care from fundholding to primary care groups, putting the commissioning of care into the hands of all practices rather than just a few. The 'purchaser–provider split' was maintained, separating the providers of care (usually hospitals) from the purchasers of care (the PCGs and health authorities). Such health reforms aim to improve the quality of NHS care by giving primary care providers real purchasing and negotiating power with the hospital trusts.

The recently constituted National Institute for Clinical Excellence (NICE) and Commission for Health Improvement (CHI) represent an important managerial tool for improving quality. Their remit is to review treatments and therapy within the NHS, comment on their efficacy and cost-effectiveness, and ensure that standards of care continue to improve. CHI may yet be seen as a potent tool in enforcing change within organisations. Together, NICE and CHI provide the government with significant institutional means for making progress towards its stated goal of providing uniformity of care throughout the country.

Patients and quality

It has been suggested that patients are *'definers of quality, targets of quality assurance, and reformers of care'*.[21] At present, however, patients are not greatly involved in healthcare quality systems. Doctors and managers have generally found it difficult to involve them. They have been concerned that those they consult will only represent specialised interests, that they will have an axe to grind, or that they will prove to be just doctor or manager 'bashers'. The implementation of clinical governance now provides an opportunity for proper patient involvement.

Irvine[22] lists patient expectations with regard to their doctors in the following terms (*see* Box 9.5).

Box 9.5:   What patients expect from their doctors[22]

- Good communication
- The ability to make their own decisions about management options
- Lack of medical arrogance
- Professional confrontation of poor practice
- Increased professional accountability
- Professional toughness in the face of malpractice or misconduct

---

Recent work has introduced the concept of a 'patient-generated index'.[23] This measures how patients feel that their illness impacts upon their daily lives. Although early work suggests that this may be a useful tool, it will need to be made more acceptable and meaningful to patients. It potentially gives them the opportunity to become more fully involved in decision making which might affect their quality of life, and for the elements of this quality to be more clearly defined. Berwick, in a forward look at the NHS,[24] recognises the importance and value of patients being able to make informed decisions about their future.

Patients have statutory representation within the NHS through Community Health Councils (which are to be replaced by advocacy services). Their work tends to focus on complaints (i.e. unacceptable care) rather than on the development of improved care. A few general practices have patient participation groups as a means of obtaining patient input.

Is there a place for quality assurance?

Going beyond the notion of quality or audit, the question arises as to whether there is a place for quality assurance. Would such assurance serve to regulate or to improve? Should it be assurance or assessment? Is there a need for quality control rather than assessment? Two contrasting approaches to quality assurance in healthcare have been suggested by Don Berwick.[25]

The first is a regulatory function, namely *quality by inspection*, with the aim of finding the 'bad apples' and rooting them out. Clearly this can engender hostility and defensiveness among those who are being inspected. However, the strength of such an approach is that it offers defined, external standards applied by a body that is not involved in the actual provision of care. This brings with it public approval and some guarantee of the level of performance. Contractual and statutory arrangements would be inspected in this way. Within medical education, the process of summative assessment at the end of postgraduate training for general practice is one form of inspection. It sets out a minimum standard, but it is both complex and a substantial consumer of time and money. Moreover, it only seeks to identify the tiny percentage of trainees whose standards are deficient.[26]

Berwick's second approach to quality assurance is that of *continuous improvement*. This assumes that the majority of practitioners wish to do a good job and that, through learning and co-operation, they will indeed continue to improve. This positive approach to quality assurance finds support in the management literature.[27,28] The hope is that clinical governance will in general follow this latter route.

Over recent years many general practices have embraced the ideal of quality, and have used various external measures as indicators of quality-assured care. A number of evaluation packages have been developed. Some of these, like the King's Fund Organisational Audit, are just that – a method of looking at systems of care and their organisation, rather than the care itself.[29] Others, like the Royal College of General Practitioners' Quality Practice Award, also include measures of clinical care.

Leadership

In all quality improvement programmes – and that is what clinical governance is – leadership is a vital ingredient.[30] Most of us are not born leaders but learn to lead because we have to. Leadership remains a widely misunderstood role. The traditional picture is of a person who is 'special', who makes key decisions and who energises the troops. A more realistic and useful image of the leader is a person with a more subtle role, who challenges prevailing models, fosters new patterns of thinking and builds a shared vision. Schein describes the leader as one who *'builds an organisational culture and shapes its evolution.'*[31]

General practice – and general practitioners – tend to distrust leaders. In recent years, some practices have developed the role of executive partner. This person has significant management roles. However, the traditional management structure in a practice is a 'flat' one, in which the partners reach a consensus,[32] and this remains the model for most practices.

It is important for the profession of general practice to appreciate that the term 'leader' does not necessarily mean 'boss'.[33] The leader helps the partnership to define its strategic aims and to achieve them. The leader also ensures the development of the team through education. Recent evidence suggests that the leadership skills of general practitioners and clinical governance leads vary greatly.[34] One of the challenges for the profession posed by clinical governance is the recognition and development of leadership within practices and groups.

Professions and self-regulation

Clinical governance is associated with lifelong learning and professional self-regulation. Johnson defines professions as having:[35]

- a professional knowledge base
- a social control of expertise
- a wish to protect clients from incompetence and exploitation.

To facilitate this, professions have codes of conduct, an orientation to service and an emphasis on moral probity. The professions also conduct careful recruitment and training, and have codes of ethics, and committees to deal with breaches of these[36] (*see* Chapter 3). Through these factors professions gain status. Successful implementation of clinical governance is a key factor in maintaining the privilege of self-regulation.

Under-performance

Professionals should have personal mechanisms to monitor their performance. If specific advice on performance is required, the local GP tutor should be able to help. The size of the problem of significant under-performance, and its management, have been discussed elsewhere.[37,38]

The recent discussion document from the Chief Medical Officer, *Supporting Doctors, Protecting Patients*,[39] has introduced the possibility of suspension of GPs whose practice is in doubt, the development of a tighter managerial role in areas that are classically perceived as being professional, and the concept of assessment centres. These were to be places where doctors whose competence was in question would be assessed. Most of the bodies involved believe that what is more important is not theoretical competence, but rather professional practice in the workplace.

A major need that has not been addressed either by this discussion document or by the profession itself is the placement of doctors who have been found to be seriously under-performing. There will be a need for theoretical and practical retraining, but also for a sheltered environment in which these doctors can re-enter practice. This demands both specific funding and specialised practices that are able to provide the level of supervision that will reassure patients that they are receiving adequate care.

Conclusion

Clinical governance is a concept in the process of development. However strong the desire for quality improvement might be, such improvement can only flourish if the environment (or culture) is responsive to the quality agenda. And there is still the issue of how to tackle poor performers and poor performance in the healthcare setting.

Summary points

- Ten key components (commandments) of clinical governance have been identified.
- Primary care organisations are responsible for implementing clinical governance.
- Quality is widely discussed but difficult to measure.
- It is vital to promote a 'quality environment'.
- Patients have a right to be involved in the quality debate.
- Poor performance can no longer be ignored.

References

1   Buetelow SA and Rowland M (1999) Clinical governance: bridging the gap between managerial and clinical approaches to quality of care. *Qual Health Care.* **8**: 184–90.

2   Secretary of State for Health (1997) *The New NHS: Modern, Dependable.* HMSO, London.

3   Secretary of State for Health (1998) *A First-Class Service: Quality in the New NHS.* Department of Health, London.

4   Royal College of General Practitioners (1999) *Clinical Governance: Practical Advice for Primary Care in England and Wales.* Royal College of General Practitioners, London.

5   'The degree to which patient care services increase the probability of desired patient outcomes and reduce the probability of undesired outcomes, given the current state of knowledge.' Joint Commission on the Accreditation of Health Care Organisations (1989) *Quality Assurance in Managed Health Care Organisations*. JCAHO, Chicago.

6   'Providing care of the highest quality *whilst* providing this at the lowest possible cost.' Donabedian A (1980) The definition of quality: a conceptual exploration. In: *Explorations in Quality Assessment and Monitoring*. Health Administration Press, Ann Arbor, MI.

7   Thus Donald Irvine offers (1) quality assessment, (2) professional development, (3) practice management and teamwork and (4) accountability, incentives and resources. Irvine D (1990) Standards in general practice: the quality initiative revisisted. *Br J Gen Pract*. **40**: 75–7.

8   Eraut M (1994) *Developing Professional Knowledge and Competence*. Falmer Press, London.

9   Secretary of State for Health (1989) *Working for Patients*. HMSO, London.

10 Marinker M (1990) Principles. In: M Marinker (ed.) *Medical Audit and General Practice*. BMJ Books, London.

11 Grilli R *et al.* (2000) Practice guidelines developed by speciality societies: the need for a critical appraisal. *Lancet* **355**: 103–6.

12 Early views obtained from managers on clinical governance revealed, among a number of factors, the hope that clinical governance would increase accountability and develop systematic quality. Patients' representatives looked for similar developments, whilst chairs of primary care groups recognised the development of quality as an aim, along with professional development. Taylor G B (2000) Clinical governance in primary care: early views of involved groups. *J Clin Govern*. **8**: 5–11.

13 Pringle M, Bradley C and Carmichael CM (1995) *Significant Event Auditing: a Study of the Feasibility and Potential of Case-Based Auditing in Primary Medical Care*. Occasional Paper No. 70. Royal College of General Practitioners, London.

14 Education Committee for General Practice (1998) *Criteria for the Appointment and Reappointment of Trainers*. Postgraduate Institute for Medicine and Dentistry, Newcastle upon Tyne.

15 Jelley D and van Zwanenberg T (2000) Peer appraisal in general practice: a descriptive study in the Northern Deanery. *Educ Gen Pract*. **11**: 281–7.

16 Hearnshaw H, Baker R and Cooper A (1998) A survey of audit activity in general practice. *Br J Gen Pract*. **48**: 979–81.

17 Kammerling RM and Kinnear A (1996) The extent of the two-tier service for fundholders. *BMJ*. **312**: 1399–401.

18 Keeley D (1997) General practice fundholding and health care costs. *BMJ*. **315**: 139.

19 Audit Commission (1994) *General Practitioner Fundholding in England*. HMSO, London.

20 Audit Commission (1996) *Fundholding Facts: a Digest of Information About Practices Within the Scheme During the First Five Years*. HMSO, London.

21 Donabedian A (1992) Quality assurance in health care: consumers' role. *Qual Health Care*. **1**: 247–51.

22   Irvine D (1999) The performance of doctors: the new professionalism. *Lancet*. **353**: 1174–7.

23   Ruta D, Garratt AM and Russell IT (1999) Patient-centred assessment of quality of life for patients with four common conditions. *Qual Health Care*. **8**: 22–9.

24   Berwick D (1998) The NHS: feeling well and thriving at 75. *BMJ*. **317**: 57–61.

25   Berwick D (1989) Continuous improvement as a sounding board in health care. *NEJM*. **1**: 53–6.

26   JCPTGP (1999) *A Guide to Certification*. JCPTGP, London.

27   McGregor D (1990) *The Human Side of Enterprise*. McGraw Hill, New York.

28   Ouchi WG (1981) *Theory Z: How American Business can Meet the Japanese Challenge*. Addison Wesley, Reading, MA.

29   King's Fund (1996) *Organisational Audit* (2e). King's Fund, London.

30   Irvine D and Irvine S (1996) *The Practice of Quality*. Radcliffe Medical Press, Oxford.

31   Schein E (1985) *Organisational Culture and Leadership*. Jossey Bass, San Francisco, CA.

32   Irvine D (1990) *Managing for Quality in General Practice*. King's Fund, London.

33   Plsek P (1999) Leadership for quality in general practice. In: *WONCA Europe '99*. WONCA, Palma, Mallorca.

34   Taylor GB (2000) Clinical governance leads: expectations and personal needs. *J Clin Govern*. **8**: 11–16.

35   Johnson TJ (1972) *Professions and Power*. Macmillan, London.

36   Rueschemeyer D (1983) Professional autonomy and the social control of expertise. In: R Dingwall and P Lewis (eds) *The Sociology of the Professions: Doctors, Lawyers and Others*. Macmillan, London.

37   Taylor GB (1998) Underperforming doctors. *BMJ*. **316**: 1705–8.

38   Taylor GB (2000) Tackling poor performance. In: T van Zwanenberg and J Harrison (eds) *Clinical Governance in Primary Care*. Radcliffe Medical Press, Oxford.

39   Department of Health (1999) *Supporting Doctors, Protecting Patients*. Department of Health, London.

CHAPTER TEN

Flexible working

Jamie Harrison

I want nothing less than the reinvention of the NHS.

Secretary of State for Health

This chapter describes how the roles of health professionals and patterns of work are changing, and it explores the concept of flexibility within primary care.

Introduction

In announcing significant extra funding for the NHS in the year 2000 and beyond, the Prime Minister warned that professionals would have to be more flexible in order to bring about the desired modernisation of the health service. Indeed, the term 'modernisation' challenges the belief that all is well in the NHS. Nowhere is this more evident than in the world of interprofessional relationships. Nurses, in particular, are challenging the status quo and widening their role to include aspects of the work of the traditional GP.

At the same time, the make-up of the general practice work-force itself is changing. The majority of medical students are women, and young doctors, both male and female, are looking for greater career opportunities. As the sociologist Isobel Allen puts it:

Medicine is no longer staffed by men working full-time in one speciality for 40 years.[1]

The wider world of work is altering rapidly, too, with increases in part-time contracts, job-sharing, teleworking and other flexible employment options. The NHS has been slow to change, but is now being forced to catch up. Inevitably what is happening in society at large impacts on traditional ways of pursuing a medical career.

The one thing we know for sure about the NHS of the future is that it will be different from now ... the NHS is an inflexible employer at a time when flexibility is important.[2]

Equally, young doctors are unwilling to wait for the NHS to change. They set their own agenda, looking beyond traditional models of immediate full-time partnership after vocational training. They travel and do locums for a year or so, look for supportive salaried posts and go where the opportunities are maximal. To borrow a phrase from management guru Charles Handy, many have decided that what they want to develop is a 'portfolio career'.[3,4]

Flexibility

If the term 'modernisation' has been overused, so has the word 'flexibility', and flexibility can have many meanings (see Box 10.1).

Box 10.1:   The meanings of flexibility

- Job substitution (e.g. nurses doing what doctors have traditionally done)
- Job development (e.g. GPs becoming more specialised within their practices)
- Different types of contracts (e.g. salaried posts in PCTs and Personal Medical Services (PMS) pilot schemes)
- Family-friendly work patterns (e.g. ability to work sessions to suit domestic needs)
- Greater patient access (e.g. longer surgery opening hours)

The aim of such 'flexibility' is to produce more efficient and effective patient care by developing the capabilities and capacity of the work-force. Pursuing such a course has its drawbacks, as it risks destabilising those members of the clinical team for whom such change is perceived as a threat to their professional values. GPs in particular find it difficult to relinquish traditional roles, even when they understand the potential benefits to them in terms of reduced workload and improved patient care.

Historically, differences between doctors and nurses in terms of power, perspective, education, pay, status, class, and (perhaps above all) gender have all too often led to what has been described as 'tribal warfare' rather than peaceful coexistence. Yet they work side by side trying to achieve the same overall end, namely an improvement in patients' health. And where GPs and nurses work together effectively, the outcomes benefit all concerned.[5]

Job substitution

Increasingly, practice nurses deal with minor injuries, prescribe basic medications and assess minor ailments, in addition to running 'well person' and disease management clinics. A recent multicentre study in South-East England of a nurse-run minor illness service demonstrated the success of this service. Patients' satisfaction with nurse consultations was greater than that for consultations with the doctor, and the number of prescriptions written, the number of patients who returned to the surgery, and the clinical outcomes later reported by patients were similar for both sets of clinicians. The only critical comment was that no attempt was made to analyse in detail the content of the consultations.[6]

Indeed, nurse involvement and expertise in general practice flourished following the 1966 Family Doctor's Charter (which encouraged the employment of practice nurses) and again after the 1990 GP Contract (which opened up nurse-led disease management clinics). One specific and more recent development has been the evolution of the nurse practitioner role in primary care (see Box 10.2).

Box 10.2:   RCN definition of a nurse practitioner[7]

An advanced level clinical nurse who through extra education and training is able to practise autonomously, making clinical decisions and instigating treatment decisions based on those decisions, and is fully accountable for her own practice.

In one study in primary care, nurse practitioners were shown to be as effective as GPs in managing 'same-day' consultations in terms of resolution of symptoms and concerns, while they provided more patient satisfaction and a longer consulting time, and gave the patients more detailed information than the GPs had done.[8] The nursing role in primary care is set to continue to change. The Secretary of State for Health had no doubt about the way in which he hoped things would develop in the future (see Box 10.3) when he talked of 'liberating nurses, not limiting them'.

Box 10.3:   The Health Secretary's 10-point challenge on nursing skills[9]

- Order diagnostic investigations, such as pathology tests and X-ray examinations.
- Make referrals to, for example, therapists and pain consultants.
- Admit and discharge patients for specified conditions and with agreed protocols.
- Manage their own patient caseloads (e.g. for diabetes or rheumatology).
- Run their own clinics (e.g. for ophthalmology or dermatology).
- Prescribe medicines and treatment.
- Carry out a wide range of resuscitation procedures, (e.g. defibrillation and intubation).
- Perform minor surgery and out-patient procedures.
- Use computerised decision support to triage patients to the most appropriate health professional.
- Take a lead in determining the way in which local health services are organised and run.

The Secretary of State for Health pointed out that nurses were already doing many of these tasks, and he expected that, with proper training, the rest would follow. Underlying this thinking is the realisation that nurses are better than doctors at doing certain things (e.g. following protocols), and that patients appreciate time spent with them by an interested therapist. Nurses may also prove to be cheaper,[10] and more malleable to NHS performance management.

Job development

What is claimed to be the philosophy which underlies much of the government's modernisation agenda – that of empowering practitioners – has been described elsewhere:

> *Modernisation requires an end to the traditional demarcations which have inhibited streamlined care for patients. There has been a vicious cycle where the NHS has not managed to perform at its full potential because it has failed to empower staff to perform to their full potential. Highly skilled nurses prevented from prescribing for common conditions because that was the traditional role of the GP. Highly skilled GPs prevented from gaining direct access to diagnostic tests because that was the preserve of hospital doctors.*[11]

Empowerment encourages a willingness to take the initiative, develop new skills and open up previously hidden horizons. In this way, flexibility ushers in an approach to providing innovative services in primary care through job development. As part of the modernisation process, some health professionals find themselves doing jobs for which they were never initially trained. Others realise the possibilities that are provided by greater specialisation of role. Box 10.4 highlights such issues.

Box 10.4:   Job development and modernisation

- Doctors and nurses manage and lead PCGs and PCTs.[12]
- Nurses manage and lead PMS pilot schemes, employing GPs and others.[13,14]
- GPs sub-specialise within their enlarging practices.[15]
- Nurses act as the first contact point for all practice patients.[16]
- Clinicians and patients use computers to share decision making in 'triadic' consultations.[17]
- Receptionists take blood samples and run a bereavement protocol.[18]

Different sorts of contracts

Along with new jobs come new contracts. The Primary Care Act Pilot (PCAP) initiatives, now more often termed Personal Medical Services (PMS) pilots, open up possibilities for flexible contracting by primary care with the NHS. The traditional terms of service whereby individual GPs contract for General Medical Services (GMS) through the Red Book regulations are set aside.[14,19]

Increasingly, young GPs are seeking alternatives to traditional GP principal posts, at least initially. Many of them opt to become locums. For others, salaried jobs appear attractive, as does the option to work part-time, especially where a work portfolio combines time spent in clinical attachments with education, research, teaching and management. This theme is reflected in the immediate career expectations of today's GP registrars (*see* Box 10.5).[20]

Primary care groups and trusts seek to appoint salaried doctors to provide 'back-fill' for their medical staff who are engaged in management and commissioning roles. Where such jobs provide ongoing support, education, training and personal and professional development, they attract large numbers of GP applicants.[21] Ordinary locum work is an attractive alternative, at least for a time, offering a different type of flexibility – significant autonomy (with regard to where and when work is done) and good pay.

Box 10.5:   Immediate career plans of 92 GP registrars on leaving their training[20]

Partnership as soon as possible	19%
GP locum	39%
Further hospital training	13%
Salaried 'career-start' post	21%
Other	8%

Nevertheless, most GPs do become principals, and the majority of those who leave a post-vocational training 'career-start' scheme join a partnership within five years.[22] More attractive salaried positions, with contracts of at least three years' duration, better pay and more say in how the organisation operates might change this situation in the near future.

Family-friendly work patterns

The government is committed to encouraging family-friendly patterns of work for NHS staff. Indeed, this is a key plank in their strategy to optimise the contribution of the workforce, not least in terms of retaining highly trained health professionals for the future:

Every NHS organisation will be judged on the flexibility they offer to staff, family-friendly working and modern training practices. If the NHS is going to compete successfully in a full employment labour market it has, as a matter of urgency, to help staff to better balance their working lives and their family lives.[11]

The 1999 extension of the Doctors' Retainer scheme to allow GP retainees to spend up to four clinical sessions per week in general practice (the previous maximum had been two) has mainly benefited women with family commitments. In addition, such doctors can carry out limited non-general medical services work by agreement with the local director of postgraduate general practice education.[19]

The government's desire to encourage evening and weekend opening of surgeries has been welcomed by some doctors as an answer to their childcare needs, since spouses and other relatives may be better placed to help domestically outside normal working hours.[23] This flexibility has naturally been challenged by those who see the working day in more traditional terms.

Job-sharing and part-time working have been the norm among practice reception staff for many years, and are now increasingly popular options across a wider spectrum of those who work in primary care. Practices have started to acknowledge this trend. Advertisements for new partners or assistants now routinely make reference to the fact that 'applicants interested in job share, full- and part-time commitments' are welcome.[24] The realisation that the job market is changing also raises concerns about who will co-ordinate the clinical work of the practice, and its practitioners, if no single clinician is regularly available on a daily basis to oversee the work. This issue is not easily resolved. Practice managers might rightly feel that clinical supervision is outside their professional remit. Nurse-led practices offer one alternative model of supervision. Another would be to develop computer-based clinical systems that are robust enough not to require such daily oversight.

Initiatives within health authorities to support primary care workers in general, and GPs in particular, play a part in improving the atmosphere and sense of well-being of those working in the service. For example, County Durham Health Authority has established a series of such initiatives under the umbrella of their NHS Beacon Service 'More scope in County Durham' (*see* Box 10.6).

Box 10.6:   'More scope in County Durham'[25]

- GP Career Start – a two-year salaried scheme for young GPs
- GP Practice Match – a mechanism to link GPs to job opportunities
- GP Choices – an occupational health-type scheme (now extended to all in primary care)
- GP Sabbaticals – a six-week opportunity for a paid locum
- GP Research and Education Fellowships – options to undertake further study and research

---

Greater patient access

As has already been mentioned, improving patient access to primary care services is fundamental to government policy, and has been so (irrespective of which government was in power) for the last ten years or more. With better access comes greater pressure to provide a more comprehensive service. Opening surgery buildings for longer periods could be more efficient (utilising otherwise dormant capacity) but it might be more costly in terms of staff provision, heating and lighting, and security issues. Inevitably those extra costs will need to be absorbed into practice budgets.

Nevertheless, some doctors welcome the opportunity to see patients outside traditional opening times,[23] and patients, particularly commuters, value such a change. For general practice to remain credible in an age of consumerism, certain shifts with regard to how and when services are provided are seen as inevitable. Yet this greater accessibility challenges notions of continuity, not least with practitioners who wish to maintain their present balance between hours worked and time to relax and be refreshed. It has also been suggested that patients could be registered with more than one practice, and thereby be able to choose the best appointment option available at the time and place required.

Conclusion

The aim to improve the flexibility of employment practices within general practice can be broadly welcomed. After all, the NHS has traditionally been an inflexible employer and, as such, it may have driven away many potential employees. The new generation of young professionals is looking for such flexibility.

However, some professionals will need to be persuaded of the wisdom of breaking down professional boundaries so quickly and risking destabilisation of the equilibrium of already hard-pressed practitioners. After all, good fences make good neighbours, and a clear understanding of roles is necessary if teamwork is to be maximised. Good leadership is clearly essential in this area, as it is always difficult to manage change well. The encouragement and development of such leaders remains a significant challenge.[12]

Summary points

- The extra funding for the NHS is conditional on health professionals demonstrating greater flexibility.
- The term 'flexibility' has several meanings, which relate to the work that professionals do (both individually and together) and the way in which they do it.
- Greater flexibility among professionals is intended to improve patient care and make services more accessible.
- Different employment options are welcome.
- Changing professional roles will be more difficult.

References

1 Allen I (1996) Careers preferences for doctors. *BMJ.* **313**: 2.

2 Carnall D and Smith R (1996) Careers advice for doctors. *BMJ.* **313**: 3.

3 Harrison J and van Zwanenberg T (eds) (1998) *GP Tomorrow.* Radcliffe Medical Press, Oxford.

4 Handy C (1996) *Beyond Certainty.* Arrow Business Books, London.

5 Salvage J and Smith R (2000) Doctors and nurses: doing it differently. *BMJ.* **320**: 1019–20.

6 Shum C, Humphreys A, Wheeler D *et al.* (2000) Nurse management of patients with minor illnesses in general practice: multicentre, randomised controlled trial. *BMJ.* **320**: 1038–43.

7 Royal College of Nursing (1989) *Nurse Practitioners in Primary Health Care – Role Definition.* Royal College of Nursing, London.

8 Kinnersley P, Anderson E, Parry K *et al.* (2000) Randomised controlled trial of nurse practitioner care for patients requesting 'same day' consultations in primary care. *BMJ.* **320**: 1043–8.

9 Milburn A (2000) speaking at the Royal College of Nursing Annual Congress in April 2000.

10 Venning P, Durie A, Roland M *et al.* (2000) Randomised controlled trial comparing cost-effectiveness of general practitioners and nurse practitioners in primary care. *BMJ.* **320**: 1048–53.

11 Milburn A (2000) speaking at the Human Resources in the NHS Conference in Birmingham on 29 February 2000.

12 Harrison J (2000) Developing leaders. In: T van Zwanenberg and J Harrison (eds) *Clinical Governance in Primary Care.* Radcliffe Medical Press, Oxford.

13 Jones D (1999) Nurse-led PMS pilots. In: R Lewis and S Gillam (eds) *Transforming Primary Care.* King's Fund, London.

14 Community Health South London NHS Trust (2000) Advert for a salaried GP at the Edith Cavell Practice – a nurse practitioner led pilot. *BMJ.* Classified Suppl. 18 March.

15 Lipman T (1999) Shifting professional roles in the primary health care team. In: T Coffey, G Boersma, L Smith and P Wallace (eds) *Visions of Primary Care.* New Health Network, London.

16 Wilson AE (2000) The changing nature of primary health care teams and interprofessional relationships. In: P Tovey (ed.) *Contemporary Primary Care. The Challenges of Change.* Open University Press, Buckingham.

17 Purves I (1998) The changing consultation. In: J Harrison and T van Zwanenberg (eds) *GP Tomorrow.* Radcliffe Medical Press, Oxford.

18 As occurs, for example, at Cheveley Park Medical Centre in Durham.

19 Harrison J (2000) Employed general practitioners. In: M Baker and R Chambers (eds) *A Guide to General Practice Careers.* Royal College of General Practitioners, London.

20 Taylor G (2000) Career plans of a cohort of GP Registrars in the Northern Deanery. *Educ Gen Pract.* **11**: 339.

21 Morley V (1999) Scheme provides regular clinical cover for PCG duties. *Prim Care Rep.* **1**: 14.

22 Delacourt L (2000) quoted in *GP* Magazine: 21 April.

23 Viney R (2000) quoted in *GP* Magazine: 28 April.

24 Dales NHS Primary Care Group (2000) Advert for salaried doctor. *BMJ.* Classified Suppl. 18 March.

25 Redpath L and Harrison J (2000) GP principal recruitment and retention in County Durham: a comparison of joiner–leaver surveys from 1996 and 1999. *Educ Gen Pract.* In press.

PART 3

The future

CHAPTER ELEVEN

What patients expect from their doctor

Laura Stroud

Fifty years of a free NHS, undistorted by fees, have indeed taught our profession to know better not than our patients, but than we ourselves once did. We have learnt that we can't produce health, healthier births, lives, and deaths by ourselves, ... or without co-operative patients constraining their personal demands within what they themselves can see, through streetwise experience, as the limits of what real communities can afford.

Julian Tudor Hart[1]

This chapter explores what patients are looking for from their GPs. Although the world is changing, certain key values persist, and there is still a clear place for the role of the family doctor.

Introduction

The ideas that inform this chapter arise from my experience – both as chair of a community health council (CHC)[*] and as a participant in various strategic and decision-making bodies in my local health system – gained as an unpaid 'volunteer'. Such participation has doubtless empowered and enriched me, yet in return I have given freely of my time, not only because I am convinced that a lay perspective in healthcare decision making is

---

[*]Although CHCs are due to be abolished (as part of the national NHS plan), the relationships and links with patient-led organisations need to be fostered and encouraged with whatever bodies replace the functions of the CHC.

important, but also because I believe that the ability of citizens to participate in the structures of a democratic society is an important right.

But why begin by establishing my credentials as a member of a CHC? Surely this is a strange opening for a chapter aimed at GPs, given that so many perceive CHCs to be 'the enemy'? After all, until recently GPs and CHCs were most likely to make contact during a formal complaints procedure, in which an officer from a CHC acts as the 'patient's friend'. Indeed, as recently as 1999, Jain and Ogden[2] found such encounters to be bruising experiences for doctors, perceiving the CHC's activity as inflammatory. However, it should be remembered that the role of the CHC goes far beyond dealing with complaints. A more positive view of CHCs would be to consider them as a conduit between health services and their local communities. Unfortunately, as a result of the independent contractor status of GPs, there has been little opportunity in the past for CHCs to work proactively with primary care providers, so it is perhaps not surprising that GPs in general have a negative perception of CHCs.

However, the world is changing. All of the NHS policy initiatives issued since the election of the New Labour government in 1997 contain powerful statements about the importance of involving patients and the public in healthcare decision making, and these have opened up opportunities for more constructive relationships between GPs and patient representatives, including CHCs. Indeed, public involvement is enshrined as one of the six key principles underlying the changes proposed in the White Paper *The New NHS: Modern, Dependable*:

> *and sixth, to rebuild public confidence in the NHS as a public service, accountable to patients, open to the public and shaped by their views.*[3]

Primary care groups (PCGs) are one of the mechanisms by which the government aims to modernise the NHS, and patient and public involvement in PCGs is a key aspect of their accountability structure. The expertise of CHCs in knowing their local communities has been of benefit to many a PCG struggling to meet the agenda set for it. I myself have sat on a selection panel interviewing prospective lay representatives for a PCG, and indeed many lay representatives on PCGs are former CHC members. CHCs have provided, almost on tap, a readily available source of advice on how to address the public involvement component of the PCG agenda, and this has done much to improve relationships. GPs and CHCs have started to work together, breaking down some of the traditional barriers that existed between them. These new working relationships have enabled each to harness the expertise that the other has to offer in order to improve the delivery and planning of healthcare services.

As an example of how patient-led organisations can work with other NHS bodies, I shall describe the results of a research project that was undertaken jointly between a trust and a CHC. A few years ago, in response to the perception held by staff in a local trust that a significant number of patients were presenting 'inappropriately' to Accident and Emergency (A and E) services, members and officers of North Tyneside CHC undertook a research project to examine the reasons why these non-urgent cases were attending the A and E department.[4] One of the key findings was that, although a proportion of the patients who presented to A and E services could have been dealt with more satisfactorily by other parts of the system, in almost every case these patients had made a rational decision to attend A and E, and had for the most part already sought advice about that decision from another professional (e.g. teacher, nurse, receptionist or even GP). The basic problem was that patients had no other timely means of accessing appropriate medical advice, especially outside normal GP surgery hours. To address this problem, the trust introduced nurse-led triage into a non-urgent minor injuries stream, independent of normal A and E services.

More generally, in order to prevent inappropriate use of expensive emergency services, it is necessary to provide more appropriate alternatives such as walk-in centres and *NHS Direct*, so that patients can access the services they want when they need them. The traditional model of GP surgery hours no longer meets the needs of patients, and this is recognised by the BMA's report, *Shaping Tomorrow: Issues Facing General Practice in the New Millennium*.[5]

As we have seen, the reform of primary care is a key part of the government's modernisation agenda for the NHS, but to understand why this is so and why patient and public participation is important, it is necessary to go back to the origins of the NHS and examine some of the tensions that arose as a result of the medical profession's reluctance to participate in the setting up of a publicly funded service. These tensions shaped the NHS that we have today, and they are responsible for some of the structural problems that the government is now trying to address.

Politics and all that ...

The NHS as an institution is over 50 years old, and many of its structures date back to the 1950s (or even earlier). In particular, the service patterns in primary care are historical – a result of the compromises that were made with the medical profession in order to gain their co-operation with the new service. Hospital consultants understood that they would benefit from a national service, but after an acrimonious campaign orchestrated by the BMA, GPs refused to become state employees and opted merely to contract to the service.[6,7] As a consequence of their willingness to participate in the new service, hospital consultants achieved a considerable amount of influence in determining the way in which resources were and are allocated. In contrast, despite being the main deliverers of health and healthcare, GPs have had little influence on the sharing of resources until recently. Thus the seeds for a major cause of inequality in healthcare were sown right at the start of the NHS, and these problems are only now beginning to be addressed with the formation of health improvement plans, primary care groups and trusts, and the rise of clinical governance. The NHS needs to function as a whole system, and the historical independence of GPs is no longer sustainable.

Despite these problems, the NHS has proved to be enduringly popular with the public. The founding principles of universality and service free at the point of use have proved to be remarkably resilient, despite the efforts of various governments to reform the NHS during the last 50 years or so. The common thread that runs through all debates on the

NHS is that of finance – it 'costs too much'. Regardless of whether the issue is the total cost, resource allocation or reconfiguration of services, there is usually a polarisation with government politicians on one side and the medical profession on the other. The public usually respond favourably to any shroud-waving by the medical profession, and successive governments have recognised that tinkering with the NHS carries a high political risk. This is perhaps why one of the most reforming Prime Ministers of recent years tried to reassure the electorate that the NHS was 'safe in her hands'. However, interestingly, the public perception is that the benefits of the NHS come from the doctors and nurses who provide the service, rather than from the politicians who fund it. This is ironic considering that the medical profession was originally opposed to the formation of a publicly funded health service. Nevertheless, the government of the day is always perceived by the public as rationing treatment and starving the NHS of much-needed funds, and the medical profession has never hesitated to take advantage of this fact.

In recent years, both Conservative and Labour governments have recognised this and have therefore introduced reforms aimed at reducing the power of the medical profession and increasing public participation in the NHS, so as to reduce the democratic deficit in the way in which decisions about healthcare are taken. In particular, the current government has invested much political capital in a modernising agenda for the NHS, maximising the benefits of its huge parliamentary majority and the public perception that Labour governments do better with the NHS. Regardless of how the current reforms translate into practice, one thing we can be sure of is that the first Labour government for 18 years is fully aware that it will be judged largely on how the general public views its performance in relation to the NHS.

The role of the consumer

The popularity of the NHS in general has meant that little fundamental change has yet been made to it (not withstanding the reforms of the last 20 years). However, in wider society, the changing patterns of work and leisure have given rise to different expectations about what constitutes good service. The service patterns of 50 years ago do not fit today's more sophisticated consumer of healthcare.

In the immediate post-war period when the NHS was formed, the vast majority of people were simply glad to have a service that was free at the point of use. However, today's consumer expects quality of service and value for money. Society as a whole is now much richer than it was, and 50 years after the formation of the NHS very few people remember what it was like before the NHS. People with disposable incomes are those who are most likely to vote, so if the NHS does not deliver the kind of service that they expect, then they may try to opt out, and this would put the publicly funded service at risk. Thus if we are to retain the NHS's founding principles of collectively funded care based on need rather than ability to pay, then quality of service is essential. In recognition of this, many of the current NHS reforms are based on the provision of more flexible services (although it is questionable whether increased flexibility necessarily results in better quality). Examples include *NHS Direct*, walk-in centres, sophisticated triage into minor injury and urgent care streams in Accident and Emergency departments, and so on.

Unfortunately, there is a tendency for the public (and NHS staff for that matter) to want the NHS they have always had. Consequently, they do not always appreciate the need for radical restructuring of the services which they have come to expect, especially when the restructuring involves the closure of existing services. Aphorisms such as 'No A and E, no MP' are burned on to politicians' hearts, causing those of us who wish to take a strategic view of service configuration to sigh at the inevitability of 'politics as the art of the possible'.

Achieving a balanced view

I began this chapter by stating that I am a member of a CHC – an organisation that some GPs believe exists solely in order to make life difficult for overworked doctors! Of course this is not true – one thing that is abundantly clear to anyone who is involved with an organisation such as a CHC is that most patients really value their doctors. Although CHCs may act on a complaint from a patient, they should not do so frivolously. My Chief Officer is absolutely clear that if she feels that there is no substance to a complaint, then that is the advice she will give to the complainant. Furthermore, any member of a CHC will tell you that over 80% of patients are satisfied with their doctors. This is also a finding of the recent National Patients Survey.[8] Finally, the statistics collected by my local CHC reveal that most complaints are about attitude rather than about clinical practice. This type of information is a valuable resource for practitioners because it can be used to improve the balance between 'good' and 'not so good' practice. However, it is perhaps worth briefly considering the Harold Shipman case. Shipman's patients were highly satisfied with his care on all of the indicators that we know are valued by patients. He gave ample time in consultation, undertook home visits frequently and involved himself in various community activities. Of course, despite being considered to be a 'nice doctor' by his patients, Shipman grossly abused his power. Thus his case provides a rather extreme illustration of the need to find an appropriate balance between what patients value and clinical indicators of good practice. In my experience, this is best achieved by the joint working of informed patient representatives and the professions.

The doctor–patient relationship

Trust is at the heart of the doctor–patient relationship. This relationship is unequal in that the store of professional knowledge, gained over years, is held by the doctor. However, patients have their own set of beliefs, individual constraints and particular needs for knowledge, too. With increasing amounts of information (sometimes of dubious quality) available on the Internet, patients are becoming better informed. Drug companies are also becoming increasingly sophisticated in their marketing techniques, targeting patients rather than doctors in order to create a demand for a new treatment or drug that is not always medically justified. Meanwhile, national organisations such as NICE are providing guidelines on best practice and making explicit decisions about whether to fund treatments such as Viagra. Often the task of the doctor is to decide how to weave these conflicting strands together. However, care and treatment should be decided by patients and doctors jointly, based on individual need but also set within realistic parameters. The establishment of new models of working should be a proactive process and not left to chance. We should actively foster the development of a culture of openness, shared responsibility and a recognition that resources are finite.

Unfortunately, in many places a social divide still exists between doctor and patient, although as society changes rapidly this may change too, particularly if plans for opening up access to medical training succeed. For example, my grandmother used to dress up to visit the doctor, as a measure of respect for his social standing, whereas my children (all pre-teens) are often invited to refer to their medical practitioners by their first names. Thus in the space of a couple of generations the mystique that set doctors apart has gone. My children's generation are growing up with the notion that their GP is an expert in their health matters and a source of advice, but by no means the *only* source of advice or necessarily an infallible one. Furthermore, given the current vogue for using nurses to deliver care in the NHS that has traditionally been given by doctors, even the role of the GP is perhaps becoming interchangeable with that of nurse practitioners and other healthcare professionals. But is this necessarily a good thing?

We know that patients like nurses. In February 2000 *The Independent* newspaper ran a story with the headline '*Patients prefer nurses to doctors, says* BMJ *study*', with reasons cited for this view being that nurses are '*friendlier, they have a different social standing and there aren't the same barriers there*'. Yet I would argue that doctors do have a unique role. They have expert knowledge, skills and a strong code of ethical and professional conduct. My personal belief – as a registered nurse myself – is that nurses have a complementary but not a replacement role. It might be useful to think of healthcare as a continuum, with nurse-led care at one end and medical care at the other, but with plenty of space in the middle to be negotiated depending on local circumstances and individual need, because ultimately what matters is patient-centred care. The inability of NHS planners to move GPs to under-doctored areas has long been known, and is encapsulated by Julian Tudor Hart's Inverse Care Law. If a needy part of the population is under-served by doctors, then the NHS must find alternative means to deliver care. *NHS Direct* has proved popular locally with socio-economically disadvantaged populations. Focus group findings from local action research to examine the effects of retirement in an under-doctored area of socio-economic deprivation showed that the patients who accessed *NHS Direct* valued the long algorithmic process. They felt 'listened to' and, for this group, it had circumvented 'rationing by receptionist'. In situations like this, nurse-led care might be appropriate and more empowering. For example, Labonte[9] used Habermas' Theory of Communicative Action[10] to explain how nurses were able to assist women in hostel accommodation to negotiate for themselves.

However, it is worth considering the professional differences between doctors and nurses because, if we do not do so, not only might we lose what is best about medical care, but also there is a danger of devaluing the core role of nursing – caring. Personally, I do not want my doctor to 'care' for me, in the sense that I wanted my midwife to care for me when I was pregnant. From my doctor I want information, realistic options, choices and risk assessment, I want a relationship that is built on mutual respect and trust, and I want some measure of flexibility about when and how I access this service.

Over the years that I have been with my practice, my GP and I have reached an agreement about the care that my family receives. On occasion, I expect to be able to ring for advice rather than make an appointment, in the certainty that I will be listened to and given appropriate advice. In return, my part of the bargain is that I do not abuse this privilege and I accept a measure of responsibility for such advice if I then choose not to visit the surgery. Both parties benefit from this type of arrangement, but it depends on mutual trust and respect between the doctor and the patient – exactly where that balance lies will depend on the individual patient (and doctor!). One of the disadvantages of providing more flexible types of services is that the relationship between medical practitioner and patient becomes more transient, and the benefits of establishing a long-term relationship are lost.

However, perhaps the notion of a personal relationship between GP and patient is somewhat artificial. I would gladly sacrifice the personal element provided there was a mechanism or process by which my preferences and personal constraints were known. The reality of the personal aspect is that I do not 'know' my GP any more than he 'knows' me. What he does know are those details of my personal history that impinge on my medical care. He can also make judgements about my knowledge and ability to assimilate information. But do I want the *Dr Finlay* or *Peak Practice* model of personal involvement in my life? The answer is definitely not (but then I don't live in a rural community!). By only having a superficial personal relationship with my GP, I am more free to discuss real anxieties with a professional I trust but do not know as an individual. I am confident of my doctor's professional conduct and ethical codes, and I also know that were he to breach these he would have a great deal to lose. The professional accountability of nurses is different, as it is designed to meet different purposes. If a shift from doctor-led to nurse-led primary care were to occur, then more than service patterns would change. Nurse education and training would also need to be fundamentally altered.

Opening up the closed shop

GPs sometimes feel that they are a threatened species – undervalued, under-resourced and overworked, with too many outsiders throwing bricks into the garden. On 23 February 2000, *The Times* and *The Daily Telegraph* ran the headlines '*GPs not wanted*' and '*Medics on Web force Dr Finlay to retire*' in the context of the BMA report *Shaping Tomorrow*.[5] However, if doctors feel under threat, the answer lies partly within their control – the old professional closed shop that was unhelpful at the start of the NHS is still partly in existence, keeping out 'secular interests'. However, in my experience, doctors have nothing to hide and much to be proud of.

For example, as a member of a Deanery GP Trainer Selection panel, I can and do say publicly that I am extremely impressed by the standards laid down, the robustness of vocational training and the sophisticated grasp that the prospective trainers have on what used to be called 'soft' patient issues. Moreover, some practices have developed such innovative methods of handling complaints that I use them as exemplars in talks, and so help to spread good practice. However, it is worth noting that in order to involve me in the trainer selection process, key individuals took risks to allow me to become an equal member of the panel. Some measure of professional power – in this case the right to determine solely within the profession who can become a trainer – was transferred to me as a member of the public. However, it is only from small steps such as these that we can begin to break down the patient–professional divide.

To take another example, I have recently been appointed as a lay representative to a University Medical School Board of Studies, and was delighted to read a superb document on the teaching of the patient–doctor relationship and communication skills. The new generation of practitioners is receiving a sound grounding in the theory of social medicine, and is also being given tools to enable them to develop a reflective style when in practice. Perhaps the medical profession should undertake a PR exercise to demonstrate to the public that their training processes are excellent!

To conclude ...

The NHS is alive and well but is undergoing a radical and (in my opinion) much-needed modernisation. Doctors are valued professionals who should continue the slow process of opening up their profession – society itself is more open than it was at the inception of the NHS, and some would argue that it ought to be more open still.

From what I have seen as a lay representative, the standard of medical education is very good and vocational training is exemplary. By and large the practice of medicine is rewarding and exciting. Far from being condemned to live in interesting times, this is a time when some of the old inherited problems of the NHS are being addressed and there are real opportunities to deliver care to those who most need it. However, for this to be achieved we need good working relationships – within professions, between professions but most of all with patients. Note that I do not say *partnership*. We often use this word loosely, but it would be wrong to assume that the development of partnerships is easy – far from it. True partnership is difficult, and it involves the sharing or transfer of power. Many professionals struggle with the notion of sharing power between professional groups, let alone with the laity, and for some patients partnership may be impossible – they may positively want the doctor to decide for them.

Nevertheless, co-operation between patient representatives and practitioners should facilitate a better understanding of the likely components of a sustainable healthcare system – in other words, a healthcare system that satisfies the needs of a relatively wealthy advanced democracy – and such a system should be better for both patient and practitioner.

Summary points

- Local communities need to be able to voice their views.
- Local health services must learn to respond effectively.
- Doctors and nurses have complementary roles.
- The new patients are sophisticated consumers.
- Over 80% of patients are satisfied with their doctors.
- However, doctors can no longer afford to remain within a 'closed shop'.

References

1   Hart JT (1998) Our feet set on a new path entirely. *BMJ.* **317**: 1–2.

2   Jain A and Ogden J (1999) General practitioners' experiences of patients' complaints: qualitative study. *BMJ.* **318**: 1596–9.

3   Department of Health (1997) *The New NHS: Modern, Dependable.* The Stationery Office, London.

4   North Tyneside Community Health Council (1997) *Report on Survey of Reasons for Attendance at the Accident and Emergency Department, North Tyneside General Hospital.* Community Health Council, North Tyneside.

5   Mihill C (2000) *Shaping Tomorrow: Issues Facing General Practice in the New Millennium.* British Medical Association, London.

6   British Medical Association (1998) *British Medical Journal. The NHS 50th Anniversary Edition.* British Medical Association, London.

7   Rivett G (1998) *From Cradle to Grave. Fifty Years of the NHS.* King's Fund, London.

8   Department of Health (1999) *The National Surveys of NHS Patients General Practice: 1998.* DoH, London. http://www.doh.gov.uk>/public/gpnhspres.htm

9   Labonte R (1998) Health promotion and the common good: towards a politics of practice. *Crit Pub Health.* **8**: 107–29.

10   Habermas J (1984) *The Theory of Communicative Action. Vol 1.* Heinemann, London.

CHAPTER TWELVE

A young doctor's expectations

Tina Ambury

You cannot fight against the future. Time is on our side.

William Ewart Gladstone

This chapter explores the hopes and fears of one of today's younger doctors, who look for freedom, flexibility and choice in their GP careers.

Introduction

The title of this chapter raises an immediate question. Why should the expectations of a young doctor be any different to those of any other doctor? And what makes a doctor 'young' in any case? Perhaps it is simply that there is a growing body of GPs who are unwilling to accept a way of working which they see as outdated.

In part, this may be a matter of demographics. The medical work-force is becoming 'feminised' by more female graduates. Added to this, male GPs are increasingly rejecting the full-time, whole-life work ethic.[1] Some doctors of all ages have begun to discover a common desire to work in a way that puts them much more in control of their own lives. They form a disparate group, often with more differences than similarities, but united by a conscious decision to step outside the mainstream.

These GPs are termed 'non-principals'. They include locums, assistants, retainees, deputies and salaried GPs – in fact *any* GP working in primary care in a capacity other than a GP principal. They share an expectation of the future that is best appreciated by looking at where they are and what they are doing *now*. In particular, they question the value of the traditional model of how GPs contract with the NHS – the independent contractor status (ICS) of the GP partner. For them, ICS no longer offers the benefits that inspired their predecessors (*see* Box 12.1).

Box 12.1:   'Benefit myths' of independent contractor status (ICS) that non-principals question

'ICS promotes independence in clinical and financial dealings.'
But what about ...

- National Service Frameworks?
- National Institute for Clinical Excellence guidelines and protocols?
- clinical governance?
- revalidation proposals?
- the 1990 Contract, with its introduction of targets?

'ICS allows GPs to act as the patient's advocate.'
But remember that ...

- advocacy at the primary–secondary care interface is not the sole domain of GP principals
- employee status does not remove the ability to act as an advocate – GPs in the Armed Forces cannot be forced to alter their clinical decisions about a patient.

'ICS allows GPs to act as "whistle-blowers" without being vulnerable to sacking.' [2]
Yet ...

- all NHS trusts and health authorities have policies in place to protect all staff, not just GPs, who raise genuine concerns in accordance with legislation. [3,4]

Life as a non-principal

The advantages

Being a non-principal has advantages and disadvantages both to the individuals concerned and to patients and the wider NHS. So, first of all, what are the advantages and why are they considered so important by non-principals (*see* Box 12.2)?

Box 12.2:   The benefits of life as a non-principal

- Freedom of choice
- Flexibility
- Enthusiasm
- Avoiding burnout

Freedom of choice

Young doctors would like to be able to choose when and how they work without being tied down by 'unwanted baggage'. The 'baggage' can be anything from being restricted to a single working location to the potentially crippling financial commitment that joining a partnership might entail. They also seek to engage in a variety of activities – both clinical and non-clinical, and more broadly medical and non-medical. They want to experience both work and play.

These doctors, by working in this way, seek to improve and enhance their skills and widen their outlook, with a view to becoming more rounded individuals. Such people are assets to both practices and patients. After all, a happy and contented doctor is likely to be better for everyone, especially when compared to one who is tired, frustrated or bored.

Flexibility

The health service of the future will undoubtedly be a very different organisation to the one we know today. It will need a different type of doctor – the flexible doctor. Recent changes in the NHS are already stretching such flexibility to the limit, with GPs being increasingly expected to participate in extra-clinical activities such as continuing professional development, clinical governance and revalidation, and administration and management for the primary care group.

Non-principals increasingly plug the service gaps attendant on these activities in a symbiotic relationship that involves all GPs. Indeed, this relationship is vital for the smooth working of the system. The symbiosis harnesses the inherent flexibility of non-principals' work patterns, benefiting the doctors themselves as well as everyone else in primary care.

Enthusiasm

By maintaining freedom and remaining flexible, non-principals can avoid the potentially mind-numbing drudgery that can come with non-stop general practice. The prospect of nine sessions a week seeing patients – day in, day out – can eventually sap all enthusiasm for the discipline. (I know – I tried it and almost gave up medicine altogether as a result!) However, by participating in a variety of activities – from medical politics and education to hospital practitioner posts and family planning sessions – patient contact becomes something that is treasured rather than resented. How many established GPs routinely look forward to their surgeries and expect to end their consultations on a 'high'?

Avoiding burnout

Freedom, flexibility and enthusiasm are important for the prevention of burnout. Tired or disillusioned doctors are of little use to the NHS, the patients or themselves. Their low morale can affect patient care, and they are more likely to retire early from the NHS, further negating the drive to increase recruitment and retention in general practice. Having a variety of jobs both within and outside general practice provides a welcome break from the routine and keeps the intellect active.

However, the reader should not gain the wrong impression. There are quite a few downsides, and being a non-principal is not all fun – despite the popular myths that abound (*see* Box 12.3).

Box 12.3: Myths and misconceptions surrounding non-principals

Myth: *'Non-principals are "failed" principals'*
Reality: Many non-principals are so by choice, either while looking for the right practice to join, or because they do not want the financial burden associated with a partnership. Some have no choice by virtue of 'enforced' mobility – frequent relocation caused by their spouse's job.
Myth: *'Non-principals earn more money than principals, for less work'*
Reality: The BMA's recommended rates are designed to deliver 75% of the average net remuneration of principals.[5] Although non-principals are not routinely involved in practice management tasks, most of them are happy to ensure that relevant patient-associated administration tasks are completed on the patients they see (e.g. item-of-service claims). However, they need the right tools for the job. Many practices fail to make the right forms readily available to non-principals, particularly the non-regular locums.
Myth: *'Non-principals "cherry-pick" – they see the patients but don't want to know about the management issues'*
Reality: This is true to some extent, but there has to be an upside to balance the disadvantages. Seeing patients is what doctors are trained for.

The disadvantages of being a non-principal

There are negative aspects of life as a non-principal which even the most enthusiastic ignore at their peril (*see* Box 12.4).

Box 12.4: The disadvantages of life as a non-principal

- Cash-flow problems
- Job insecurity
- Isolation
- Vulnerability

Cash-flow problems

You may be as flexible as you wish, with all the freedom in the world, but it does you no good if you cannot pay the mortgage. Being available to fill a service gap at a moment's notice is all well and good, but it could also leave you with an empty diary. The dilemma could be whether to accept this booking of a two-hour surgery (and guarantee at least some income), or whether to wait in the hope that you receive a request for a longer booking at a later date.

Accepting the short surgery could mean not being available to cover a whole week that is offered later. Waiting for the more lucrative offer carries the risk of ending up with no work booked at all. Once the session or engagement has been completed, there may be a delay before payment is received. The worst culprits in this respect are not usually fellow GPs, but NHS trusts, who put the invoice through their accounts system.

Job insecurity

Today no one can either expect or demand protected employment and a guaranteed 'job for life' – not even doctors. However, non-principals, especially itinerant locums, can quite easily become victims of job insecurity, in a way that would never happen to a GP principal. Indeed, it could be argued that the inherent flexibility and multi-skilling of non-principals are the result of trying to maintain an income from any and all means possible.

However, it should also be noted that asking for job security is not synonymous with wanting a fully salaried service. A salaried service would have implications for all, not just those whose clear desire is to remain as independent contractors.

Isolation

Moving about from one job to another and from one practice to another often serves to increase the sense of isolation which is felt by most non-principals. This isolation takes many forms – professional, clinical, educational, financial and sometimes even social.

Vulnerability

The lack of an employment contract for most non-principal work, coupled with job insecurity and isolation, heightens the feelings of vulnerability of those who work in such a non-conformist way. Most non-principals are able to manage the inevitable uncertainty which goes with the style of working. They cherish their right to choose while remaining enthusiastic about their discipline. They should not feel obliged to join the orthodox mainstream of practitioners.

Many non-principals would like to help their colleagues in this mainstream change working practices to a point where the advantages of being a non-principal are available to all, not just to a minority. To achieve this, the disadvantages of flexible working (*see* Table 12.1) would need to be minimised.

Table 12.1   The 'swings' and 'roundabouts' of flexible working

Advantages	Disadvantages
Choice – where, when, how and for whom	Danger of having no work and therefore no income
Self-employed – independent	Lack of employment rights
Employee status – guaranteed work and salary	Lack of independence – restricted to employer's wishes
Can negotiate 'fair day's pay for fair day's work'	Open to exploitation
Freedom from the financial burdens associated with partnership	Job insecurity
Time for friends and family – a 'life'!	Isolation – professional, clinical, educational

Balancing career and personal life

The 'ups' of being a non-principal are about doctors enjoying their work while still having time for a life of their own. In any case, who wants a career that means the exclusion of everything else? Critics of younger doctors see this attitude of 'having your cake and eating it' as their greatest fault, and they believe that it reflects a lack of commitment. In truth, this debate hinges on the answer to the simple question 'Do you live to work, or work to live?'.

Historically, GPs were defined by what they did, and by their place in society (see Chapter 1). The job could (and sometimes did) become overwhelming. The challenge for general practice now is to offer doctors not only a satisfying career which gives pleasure and a sense of fulfilment, but also a job with manageable levels of stress and, where possible, the avoidance of disappointment and disillusionment. Box 12.5 lists these aspirations.

Box 12.5:   The aspirations of the new GP

Career
- Work planning
- 'Committed' versus 'nomadic' styles of working
- Career as income generation

Personal life
- Family and friends
- Health and well-being

Achieving balance
- Structured career pathways in general practice
- Formal career advice
- Recognising opportunity
- Achieving the 'Holy Grail'

Career

Work planning

An essential aspect of achieving a balance between home and work is effective planning. An empty work diary affords plenty of time to do all the 'fun' things in life, but does not generate income. It can also lead to a state of panic in which all offers of work are accepted, and then the desired maximum work levels may be exceeded. Neither of these situations (too little or too much work) is career enhancing, nor will they reduce stress levels. Determined organisation coupled with a strong resolve is required to prevent either of these extremes. In today's general practice 'market-place', non-principals are generally in high demand, and the consequences of poor work planning are more likely to arise from accepting too much work than from taking on too little.

'Committed' versus 'nomadic' styles of working

Work planning within a non-principal career involves deciding either to adopt a *committed* workstyle, which involves working regularly for one particular practice (or a limited number of practices), or being *nomadic*, which involves a peripatetic style of working – usually as a locum. This is normally a balance between personal choice and opportunity. Please note that commitment to the discipline of general practice is *not* primarily about where the job is done! *Commitment is about doing the job well.*

Career as income generation

As with every other job in the twenty-first century, a career in general practice must provide for the financial needs of a doctor and his or her dependants. However, working long hours in order to gain large financial rewards can leave little time for everything else, including a personal life.

Personal life

Family and friends

No man (or woman, for that matter) is an island. Taoists[6] believe that inner peace is only achieved by finding the balance between the yin and the yang – or, in this case, the home and work. Having a flexible workstyle not only allows doctors to participate in various medical fields, but it also enables them to take time off altogether – to recharge their batteries. In modern general practice, protected time is necessary, and it should not be something that has to be squeezed in whenever there is a free moment available. A person's friends and family are there to be nurtured and enjoyed, not neglected. This intimate circle has a vital role to play. It provides joy to enrich us, it supports us in times of need, and it offers a place where we can truly be ourselves.

Health and well-being

Doctors are notoriously bad at looking after their own health,[7] yet it is vital that they should do so. The stress of modern general practice seems to be destined to exacerbate health problems, and little help is provided either for the prevention of stress-related illness or to manage it in a humane way.[8] For general practice to become a career that nurtures its members, there needs to be a properly funded, universal occupational health service to which all doctors have access.[9] At present there is the paradox of non-principals opting out of the stresses of partnership-based practice only to find new stresses of their own. They then have no access to the (albeit patchy)[10] supportive structures that are available to principals.

Achieving balance

Structured career pathways in general practice

The most important planning any doctor, regardless of age, can do is to formulate a structured career path – a path that is not so inflexible as to become a rut, yet not so formless as to have the doctor wandering aimlessly from post to post. Unfortunately, general practice has little or no career structure. The traditional pattern of working involves completing vocational training in order to attain the right to independent practice, and then joining a partnership. Anything else has to some extent been regarded with suspicion. As increasing numbers of younger doctors choose to become non-principals, alternative career paths must be developed.

Formal career advice

Choosing a career path is not something a doctor can or should do in isolation. However, it may be difficult to find someone who can help them to make an informed choice. At present there is no formal structure dedicated to providing careers advice for GPs. Course organisers may provide advice for doctors who are undertaking or have recently completed vocational training. All new principals, and a proportion of non-principals, have access to the GP tutor network. Indeed, in some parts of the country GP tutors have been appointed with a specific responsibility for non-principals. There is a need for non-principals to press for better access to this network. They should also join with others in calling for the development of a dedicated careers advisory service. This should be staffed by professionals who have had formal career advice training, rather than by senior GPs with little or no formal training in mentoring skills.[11]

Recognising opportunity

Opportunity can come in all shapes and sizes. A chance encounter in a practice or at an educational meeting often leads to a job possibility. Acting on that opportunity might have a decisive effect on a young doctor's career, and such opportunities need to be grasped as and when they arise.

Achieving the 'Holy Grail'

Balancing career with a personal life can sometimes seem like an impossible task, but is this 'Holy Grail' too much to expect (*see* Box 12.6)? It seems ludicrous that a society that demands a humanistic and caring attitude from its doctors appears bent on denying them their own humanity. Younger doctors are taking the courageous step of voicing their dissatisfaction with the status quo. They are voting with their feet, despite the significant disadvantages of non-principal work discussed above.

Box 12.6:   The 'Holy Grail' of a future general practice formal career advisory service

- Structured careers in general practice
- Universally available occupational health service
- A fair day's pay for a fair day's work
- Job security
- Protected personal time

Personal development

Change and time management

Change is inevitable, often stressful and sometimes destructive.[12] Primary care groups and trusts, with their emphasis on practice development through clinical governance, may be seen to militate against the interests of individual doctors. However, individuals will increasingly be called upon to show evidence of personal development, notably with regard to revalidation. Doctors are becoming more accountable to the public and their patients than ever before. Personal development requires doctors to identify their own professional and clinical learning needs, before acting to address those needs. All doctors will need to ensure that they maintain their skills. There is a risk that the time needed for this will be taken from their already restricted personal time. The development of flexible working and the mixed model of general practice that this promotes offers one way in which doctors could protect the time that they need for personal development.

Getting a life

The humanity of the doctor is vital to their work. Patients are people and are most satisfied when their doctors behave as people too.[13] A well-rounded doctor will be more approachable and more able to show empathy to their patients, and they may also be more able to communicate with patients in a relatively jargon-free way. All work and no play makes Jack a dull boy. It could also make him a dangerous one by virtue of his becoming burnt out (and of course this applies to Jill, too).

Conclusion

Young doctors expect the following from the future:

*   freedom
*   flexibility
*   choice.

The independent contractor model that currently predominates in general practice is too restrictive. However, most young doctors do not want the present system to be discarded entirely. What young doctors – and indeed all doctors – should want and expect is evolution, not revolution. General practice needs to evolve a more flexible, mixed model that provides a range of different contractual arrangements for doctors, whilst maintaining and cherishing all that is good about the present system.

For the majority of young doctors this simply means having real choices about their career paths. Far from being a selfish outlook, this attitude will force change and breed innovation. For which is more selfish – wanting things to be better now and in the future, or wanting things to stay the same just because that demands less effort? Young doctors have come to expect more from general practice, whilst appearing (to some) to be willing to give less in return. But is the desire to have time for both work and play such a crime?

Summary points

- Young doctors are increasingly questioning the independent contractor status.
- The benefits of being a non-principal include greater freedom of choice, flexibility and maintaining enthusiasm.
- However, non-principals also suffer cash-flow problems, job insecurity, isolation and vulnerability.
- There are ways to minimise these disadvantages, particularly through careful work planning.
- Non-principals want to make the advantages of their ways of working more generally available within general practice.
- Structured career paths, sound careers advice and an occupational health service are needed for all GPs.
- Young doctors are not lacking in commitment, but they do care about a properly balanced life.

References

1 Lambert TW and Goldacre MJ (1998) Career destinations seven years on among doctors who qualified in the United Kingdom in 1998: postal questionnaire survey. *BMJ.* **317**: 1429–31.

2 Mihill C (2000) *Shaping Tomorrow: Issues Facing General Practice in the New Millennium.* British Medical Association, London.

3 Yamey G (2000) Protecting whistleblowers. *BMJ.* **320**: 70–1.

4 Department of Health (1998) *The Public Interest Disclosure Act 1998. Whistleblowing in the NHS.* Department of Health, London.

5 Harvey P (1998) *Fees for Medical Cover in General Practice.* National Association of Non-Principals (NANP), Chichester; website http://www.nanp.org.uk/rates.htm

6 Hua-Ching N (1979) *The Complete Works of Lao Tzu.* Sevenstar Communications, Santa Monica, CA.

7 Forsythe M, Calnan M and Wall B (1999) Doctors as patients: postal survey examining consultants' and general practitioners' adherence to guidelines. *BMJ.* **319**: 605–8.

8 Schattner P (1998) Stress in general practice. How can GPs cope? *Austr Fam Physician.* **27**: 993–8.

9 Chambers R, George V, McNeill A *et al.* (1998) Health at work in the general practice. *Br J Gen Pract.* **48**: 1501–4.

10 Chambers R, Miller D, Tweed P *et al.* (1997) Exploring the need for an occupational health service for those working in primary care. *Occup Med.* **48**: 485–90.

11   Freeman R (1997) Towards effective mentoring in general practice. *Br J Gen Pract.* **47**: 457–60.

12   Haslam D (ed.) (2000) *Not Another Guide to Stress in General Practice!* (2e). Radcliffe Medical Press, Oxford.

13   Gore J and Ogden J (1998) Developing, validating and consolidating the doctor–patient relationship: the patients' views of a dynamic process. *Br J Gen Pract.* **48**: 1391–4.

CHAPTER THIRTEEN

The new GP

Tim van Zwanenberg

Chaos often breeds life, when order breeds habit.

Henry Brooks Adams

This chapter describes the challenges facing general practice, and proposes that some broad functions emerge – consumer-responsive care, care based on a relationship, 'specialist' care, and contributing to the corporate governance of primary care. Given the apparent chaos of the NHS, complexity theory may provide a better model for understanding the changes or at least accepting them with greater equanimity.

Introduction

It is clear that the life of a general practitioner has changed dramatically since 1948. At that time general practitioners had to contend with very large numbers of patients, were available at all times, and consulted and visited much more often than their modern counterparts. Although the number of patients seen, especially on home visits, is much lower today, their demands and those of society in general are qualitatively greater. Indeed, many such patients have complex mixes of long-term physical, mental and social problems.

At the same time, the status of the doctor has been somewhat diminished. There was a time when general practice was a highly respected profession and doctors regulated their own affairs. The public liked what they got (as well as being unable to choose otherwise) and general practitioners had predictable career paths and comfortable lifestyles, but now almost everything is different.[1]

With a changing pattern of work and place in society come new (and, some would argue, damaging) stresses. For example, doctors in the 1980s had longer working hours yet more stimulating work than people in other occupations. Now the picture is different, with both male and female doctors reporting increasing demands on their time, and reduced ability to control their work.[2] Furthermore, the differences between doctors and others in primary care appear to have levelled out, with most healthcare workers struggling to remain in control at work.

Challenges to general practice

For general practitioners, the forces driving change have presented them with a range of challenges which are both powerful and threatening (*see* Box 13.1). Understanding these challenges may help to distil out what it is that GPs of the future will do, and their place in the world, for it appears that patients, at least, still want to see a doctor.

Box 13.1:   The challenges to general practice

Consumerism
- Demand for easier access
- Better-informed patients
- Self-help groups
- 'Patient partnership'

Substitution
- NHS Direct
- Nurse practitioners
- Hospital outreach
- Complementary therapies
- Multiprofessional teamworking

Accountability
- Professional regulation – revalidation
- Appraisal
- Clinical governance
- Health and Safety legislation
- Employment law
- Media interest

Generational change
- Increasingly feminised work-force
- More prevalent part-time working
- Generation X values – less commitment to traditional views
- Dependence on the commitment of older doctors
- Undermining the covenant model?

The new 'managerialism'
- Modernisation
- Guidelines – National Institute for Clinical Excellence (NICE)
- National Service Frameworks (NSFs)
- Inspection – Commission for Health Improvement (CHI)
- The NHS Plan

Consumerism

The consumerist drive for access to services permeates society (*see* Chapter 2). Why, people argue, should advice about our health be any different? After all, you can now order a pizza, shop at a supermarket or withdraw money from a bank at any time, day or night. Moreover, not only do patients want better access, but they are now increasingly unwilling to accept a second-rate service. They are better informed about their rights and about their condition and its treatment. They obtain books and leaflets on health, and many of them routinely search the Internet. Self-help groups produce evidence-based information advising patients what they should expect of the health service. As a result, many patients with chronic disease are now better informed about their condition than their GP. They have become 'expert patients'.

These new generations of patients will no longer remain the passive recipients of a service, nor will they tolerate medical arrogance. Instead, some are attracted by the notion of partnership, both in individual relationships with their own doctors and in their relationship with healthcare organisations. Patient involvement in determining priorities and planning primary care services is now expected.[3]

Substitution

One of the great paradoxes that perplexes commentators is the apparent resentment by general practitioners of their workload, coupled with their resistance to delegating it to someone else. Indeed, doctors themselves appear to relish taking on greater responsibilities in research, teaching and management.

Recently, this resentment has been aimed at *NHS Direct*, which stands accused of absorbing extra resources that might have bolstered traditional services. Such negative responses tend to greet any new initiatives, such as nurse practitioners or hospital outreach services. General practitioners seem unwilling to let anyone else do 'their work'. Why should this be, and what is it that only general practitioners can do?

Equally, the societal trend towards using complementary therapies has further challenged the role of general practitioners as the main source of primary medical advice. Detractors may protest about the lack of evidence of the efficacy of such therapies (the hard evidence for the efficacy of general practitioners is hardly overwhelming), but patients continue to seek help, particularly for those intractable symptoms for which orthodox medicine has offered so little to date. A routine first appointment with a homeopathic practitioner can last for up to an hour, and patients are given time to talk. Although general practitioners do provide such time for patients to talk – on average 47 minutes a year per patient[4] – both they and their patients feel pressurised to limit the consultation time. Patients often comment 'I know you have a lot of people waiting' or 'I don't want to waste your time' or ' I know you must be very busy, doctor'. And few GPs deny being busy. Of course, in our culture, busyness is linked to status – the busier a person is, the more important they must be.

The movement towards greater involvement with other professionals has also brought its own threats. Most major current health problems are multidimensional in origin, requiring collaboration between health and social care in, for example, neighbourhood renewal or preventing unwanted pregnancies.[5] Gone are the days when the doctor's word held sway and the medical model was the norm. The new social model of disability, racial and cultural diversity and social inclusion is based on civil rights and removing barriers and discrimination. People using services are placed in an entirely different relationship with professionals. The shift is from separatism between services and patronage on the part of professions to partnership.[6]

Partnership requires new skills, yet general practitioners and other professional groups have had little relevant training in these in either their undergraduate course or their continuing professional development.[7] This is not surprising. Until recently, protecting professional identity was the key to qualification and career progression. Future measures of professional success may well include the capacity to operate across the boundaries of profession and system of care. General practitioners could find themselves ill-equipped for this new world where negotiation, conflict resolution, and understanding and managing change are all fundamental skills. There is no doubt that nurses will continue to take on increasing levels of responsibility in the monitoring and management of patients with chronic illness in primary care.

Accountability

The drive for greater accountability currently pervades much of the fabric of medicine, and was the focus of some of the earlier chapters of this book. At the basis of this is the need for greater honesty and openness about mistakes. In 1988, Julian Tudor Hart entitled the centrepiece chapter of his book, *A New Kind of Doctor*, 'A crisis of accountability'.[8] He made the point that, for the 40 years following the inception of the health service in 1948, the legal definition of GPs' work in the NHS (contained in the Regulations of the NHS Act)[9] had been:

> *to render to their patients all necessary and appropriate medical services of the type usually provided by general practitioners.*

In other words, GPs did what GPs did – defining their work and determining their own standards.

In this they had been helped by the permissive nature of the contract and payment arrangements which followed the 1966 *Charter for the Family Doctor Service*.[10] These measures increasingly fostered the formation of group practices, the employment of ancillary staff, the development of premises and an expansion in the range of services offered to patients. However, the pace of development during the two decades following the introduction of the Charter was far from uniform, and this did not go unnoticed by the government. The 1990 GP Contract was the first step in making general practitioners more accountable for what they did. At the time the government was accused of trampling on their professional autonomy and of imposing clinical direction.[11] However, the requirements of the 1990 GP contract seem quite tame compared to what is proposed now, namely annual appraisal, quinquennial revalidation and clinical governance.

It is not just general practitioners as individual doctors who are being called to account. The collegiate foundation of general practice – the partnership – is increasingly obliged to adhere to new legislation and good practice in arenas other than medicine. Practices, as small businesses, are at risk of breaching Health and Safety Regulations (e.g. in the disposal of sharps and clinical waste). They are liable for other hazards to the public which might arise from the design or use of their buildings. In the matter of employment, practices must comply with legislation on race, gender and disability discrimination. The independent contractor status may confer benefits, but it also carries with it substantial risks. In the long term it may be these that hurry GPs into larger primary care organisations which are better equipped to assess, minimise and absorb risks of all types.[12]

There are other pressures, too. Patient groups, as well as the media, are taking an increasing interest in doctors and the health service. Cases before the GMC, which might previously have warranted a few lines on the inside pages, now provoke front-page banner headlines in the newspapers. Notwithstanding certain notable exceptions, most of these cases seem to come from the hospital sector, and in general it appears that people still trust their GPs.

Generational change

Between 1988 and 1994 there was a 31% fall in the number of male doctors recruited to GP vocational training schemes in England and Wales, and a 4% rise in the number of female doctors, who by 1994 represented the majority at 55% of the total.[13] This trend towards greater numbers of women doctors in general practice has continued and will not be reversed. In some medical schools the proportion of female undergraduates in some years is as high as 85%.

This increasing so-called 'feminisation' of the work-force is accompanied by other trends. Part-time working, portfolio working and career breaks are now commonplace among both male and female general practitioners, and the new generation of young professionals appears to have different values. These members of generation X seek to achieve a better balance between home, career and recreation.[14] They perceive their older colleagues (from the baby-boomer generation) as over-committed to work.

However, many of these older doctors are going to be around for the next 20 years or so. Is their dedication to patients and the NHS, whether misplaced or not, to be taken for granted by their younger professional colleagues? Or will the younger doctors become more like their older colleagues when they in turn reach their forties? There may be comfort in identifying the things that younger doctors are not criticising, but questions remain. What must doctors retain if they are still going to be professionals? Can they discard the 'long-hours culture' and still sustain sufficiently professional relationships with patients? What must the NHS do to retain doctors?

Some consequent dangers loom. First, it is argued, from perceptions of those places where a professional work-force has become feminised, that the profession will lose social and political status. Secondly, if the new generation of doctors is less committed, what might become of covenanted relationships? Consolidating a new relationship between patients and doctors, which is for instance the prime rationale for revalidation, does depend on a very real level of commitment on behalf of both parties.

The 'new managerialism'

The government has demanded change under its programme of modernisation – change for cash, investment coupled with reform.[15] By any standards its decision to inject £19.4 billion into the NHS over the four years from the year 2000 – an annual average growth of 6.1% – was generous. Yet this generosity and the Prime Minister's personal involvement reflect, among other things, frustration at the failure to achieve the desired transformation of the NHS.[16] As part of the settlement, five modernisation action teams were established, and one of these was charged to tackle professional change. The Prime Minister himself challenged the professions to get rid of unnecessary demarcations, introduce more flexible training and working practices, and ensure that doctors did not deal with patients who could be treated safely by other healthcare staff.[17] This, coupled with the Prime Minister's perceived support for the idea that *NHS Direct* might replace general practitioners as the gatekeepers of the NHS, merely heightened GPs' crisis of identity.

It may be of some comfort to know that these types of demands are not new! In 1912, Lloyd George made the following statement when speaking in Parliament on his proposal to increase the annual payment to panel GPs:[18]

> *If the remuneration is increased, the service must be improved ... I have got three conditions which I am going to lay down as the result of this increased provision.*

However, there is other evidence that the government has become increasingly centralist in its relationship with the NHS. Witness the creation of the National Institute for Clinical Excellence (NICE), the National Service Frameworks (NSFs), the NHS Performance Framework with accompanying performance league tables, the national patients' survey, the Commission for Health Improvement, and finally the NHS Plan. And the NHS is not alone in this – the education service has been similarly affected.

It appears that this government-led 'new managerialism' is applied primarily to those services which are high on the government's list of political priorities. Greater government interest, which is not necessarily a bad thing when resources are being allocated, leads to more centralised management. The problem is how to achieve change throughout a huge organisation such as the NHS. The traditional model is that ministers decide and professionals deliver, but does this work? It has been argued that '*rather than frog-marching the NHS towards best practice, the government should be motivating professionals within the NHS to innovate, experiment and learn from each other*'.[19] General practitioners might take heed of the fact that they need to create enough space for themselves to allow innovation.

Comfort in chaos – complexity theory

Inevitably the forces which lie behind these challenges are not driving change in the same direction – far from it. Before attempting to describe where general practitioners might fit in this maelstrom, it might be worth dwelling for a moment on the theory of complexity, for that may help in understanding, or at least in accepting with some equanimity, the world around us. Complexity theory is derived from a number of disciplines and based on the notion of chaos (i.e. it recognises that many phenomena are the consequence of non-linear interactions of many and various elements – interactions that cannot be understood simply by breaking them down into their constituent parts).[20]

Complexity theory thus challenges the logic of the traditional scientific approach. Instead we have 'post-normal medicine'[21] – a holistic approach that reflects diversity, rich interaction and complex dynamics. In terms of comprehending the NHS, this must be a better basis than the typical reductionist view which divides and subdivides complex systems into ever smaller parts in order to study their properties. Once divided in this way their relevance to the whole becomes less and less apparent.

Indeed, it is arguable that health and the delivery of healthcare are much more complex than typical management theory derived from industry supposes. The human being itself is a highly complex system in which mind and body interact in ways that are still poorly understood. Small chemical changes produce large and sometimes surprising and unexpected results. So-called evidence-based medicine is probabilistic. We are not in a field of Newtonian cause and effect. Healthcare is a matter of restoring equilibrium – helping people to feel healthy. This can involve reducing their expectations with regard to their health.

A national health service is extremely complex, since it involves attempts to co-ordinate a range of resources – people, skills and facilities – around the delivery of outcomes which are themselves highly complex and not entirely specifiable. Target setting (e.g. NSFs) may therefore have its place, but ought never to be allowed to predominate, since it is inherently reductionist. One of the threats to general practice is the mistaken belief that performance in the field of health is simply a matter of applying the same techniques that might be used to study the performance of a car plant. Human beings are complex systems in a way that manufactured goods are not.

The example of birds flocking might give us a clue about the NHS. Both are complex systems with multiple interactions. It is theoretically possible to break down the forces that act on each bird in the flock into a series of mathematical equations, which can be related one to the other. Several high-grade mathematicians, a vast computer and several years' time could see the task complete. Alternatively, complexity theory, taking a holistic view, would conclude that there are a small number of rules which govern the birds' behaviour – they are all trying to get to the same place, they fly as close together as possible and they do not touch each other.

A similar analysis of the NHS might be that all behaviour is based on three 'rules':

*   the need to satisfy the patient
*   the need to satisfy the professional
*   the need to meet the priorities of the NHS (i.e. the government).

There is clearly tension in this, but it does offer the hope of a balanced equilibrium where none of these is ever paramount and none is ever irrelevant. A few simple rules may be much more effective than endless guidance. This idea incidentally mirrors the previous Chief Medical Officer's definition of continuing professional development in the NHS,[22] which recognised the tripartite interest, namely patients, professionals and the NHS. It also neatly explains why an alliance between patients and professionals is so critical at the moment in order to counterbalance the centralising power of government.

Emerging functions

Against this background of complexity and countervailing forces, a number of broad functions emerge that need to be undertaken in primary care, where GPs have a role (*see* Box 13.2), and there is likely to be a mixed economy of both patients and doctors. Patients will differ from each other in the service or individual practitioner they want, and will also make different selections at different times. (There should probably be more experimentation in this, as patients may well be highly proficient at choosing appropriately.) This 'market segmentation' is fairly obvious, and is well recognised in retail and service industries. Equally, doctors will move between different functions, changing their roles as they do so.

Consumer-responsive primary care

It is now known that many patients, in certain circumstances, are content with (and in some cases may indeed prefer) being able to seek advice from a professional with whom they do not have a prior personal relationship. General practitioners have learned this particularly from working in out-of-hours co-operatives. Patients with acute illness want easy access to a quality service, but do not have to see their own doctor. Equally, *NHS Direct* is widely used and may be the service of choice for some groups in the population (e.g. young men, who perhaps favour the more impersonal service offered by a call centre, do not want a face-to-face consultation, and also prefer to avoid having to face the practice receptionist!). Patients do not have to leave the house, and can use information technology (IT) which they prefer and are used to. Finally, they do not have to worry about 'upsetting the doctor'.

Computer-based triage, operated by nurses on the telephone, in GP out-of-hours co-operatives and in Accident and Emergency departments, may provide the most effective and satisfactory method of prioritising and 'signposting' patients out of hours. Acute

---

Box 13.2:   Emerging functions

Consumer-responsive primary care
- 24-hour access to advice
- Computer-programmed triage
- Signposting to appropriate services

Relationship-based care
- Based on the general practice consultation
- A relationship between doctor and patient
- Sorting the unsorted
- Longer-term care of the chronic and complex
- Access to a wide range of other services

'Specialist' care
- Intermediate care
- Clinical assistantship in hospital settings
- Undertaking procedures (e.g. vasectomies)
- Providing services (e.g. for substance abuse problems)
- Taking referrals (e.g. dermatology)

Corporate management of primary care
- Clinical governance
- Public health needs assessment
- Constructing guidelines and protocols
- Priority setting
- Managed care

---

problems seem to be particularly amenable to such triage. At these times general practitioners would no longer 'man the front door' of the health service. Instead they would apply their skills more appropriately to those patients who required them (e.g. patients with unsorted medical problems in need of diagnosis and initial management, directed to them by nurse-led triage).

It remains to be seen how fulfilling call-centre work is for nurses in the longer term, but this arrangement might help to protect GPs from being seen as the source of advice for all things, even non-health related matters.

Relationship-based care

Although impersonal services suit some individuals at some times, in other situations patients want a relationship with their professional attendant. This is more likely to be the case if patients want someone to listen, someone to consider their problems in depth, or if they are seeking professional judgement or support. The consultation in general practice provides the ideal vehicle for building these relationships and meeting these needs. Increasingly the relationship, once established, extends beyond the individual practitioner to the rest of the practice team.

The results of a Swedish study on patients with diabetes are of interest in this context.[23] The patients were asked how they would like decision making between themselves and their doctors to occur (i.e. who would make the decision and how) (*see* Box 13.3). Over 75% of the patients wanted the doctor to make the decision, although more than 50% wanted a discussion with the doctor first. Patients are willing to share risk but do also seek clinical judgement.

Box 13.3:   Decision making between doctors and patients with diabetes

Doctor to make decision alone	19%
Doctor to make decision after discussion with patient	57%
Patient to make decision after discussion with doctor	23%
Patient to make decision alone	1%

'Specialist' care

The considerable expansion in intermediate care and related services which focus on supporting older people in the community will inevitably involve GPs in the care of patients who would previously have been cared for in hospital. For example, rapid-response teams are intended to prevent admission, and other services are designed to hasten discharge. Many GPs will need to develop new skills and expertise in this area.

There are already many 'specialist' GPs working as clinical assistants in hospitals, and as a result of GP fundholding and other initiatives, others provide practice-based specialised services (e.g. surgical procedures such as vasectomy and endoscopy, or substance abuse services). Indeed, inter-practice referral is now commonplace in some areas, with GPs offering their colleagues an alternative source of specialist advice on diagnosis and management in areas such as dermatology, psychosexual medicine, and so on.

The traditional boundary between general practice and the specialties appears set to become more blurred, with GPs increasingly developing new 'specialist' skills to support the development of local services for patients. This trend poses a challenge to those who would prefer to restrict such practice to the realm of consultants.

Corporate management of primary care

General practitioners have been used to running their own businesses. With the advent of GP fundholding, locality commissioning and now primary care groups and trusts, many GPs have experience in NHS management beyond the practice. They have participated in decisions on limiting services as well as developing them. However, commissioning (and fundholding before it) is primarily concerned with services provided by others (i.e. hospitals). Now general practitioners involved with primary care groups and trusts have to address the quality of primary care – not only the range of services provided but also their clinical governance. They are expected to work in partnership with patients, other professionals and GPs from neighbouring practices. As if all of that were not enough, they are also charged with increasing equity and enhancing the public health – no small task.

Skills that are required of general practitioners

We have already described the range of skills required of GPs (*see* Box 13.4), including the ability to look after oneself, balance work and leisure and cope with the 'new managerialism', consultation skills for meeting patients' needs and conferring professional credibility, teamworking and the ability to work in partnership across traditional boundaries, openly demonstrating quality of care, and being able to relate to the wider public and political bodies. We also proposed three 'strategic themes' for general practice, namely *leadership* to embrace and lead change, *scholarship* for intellectual stimulation, and *fellowship* for mutual support.[24]

Box 13.4:   Skills required of general practitioners

- Managing self
- Consulting with patients
- Working with others
- Maintaining good practice
- Relating to the public

Of these, the development of leadership among general practitioners is perhaps the most pressing need. In a system predicated on peer relationships, the notion of leadership appears counter-intuitive. However, leadership is a function much needed by organisations at times of turbulence, for leaders can empower and enable others to harness and implement change. Sir Kenneth Calman said that '*leadership requires knowing where you want to go, taking people with you, and giving sufficient time and energy to make it happen*'.[25] This latter aspect of leadership, which promotes organisational development, is much needed in primary care at the moment.[26]

What do general practitioners bring?

Against this background of change and concomitant threat, it is reasonable to ask what general practitioners can 'bring to the party'. What knowledge, skills and attitudes do they possess that will be needed? With patients' increasing access to the Internet, GPs are no longer the repository of all knowledge, but they are generalists and do have breadth of knowledge. This enables them to offer judgement and the wisdom of experience. Increasingly they may take the role of interpreter in the 'triadic' consultations, where the patient tells the story, the computer provides the evidence and the doctor attempts to make sense of both for the benefit of the patient.[27] In this process they can also share risk with the patient.

The skilled general practitioner can also adjust his or her attitude to suit patients' needs. Not all patients are the same or indeed want the same. Some want quite close personal relationships, whereas others prefer more impersonal services. Some would like a more equal partnership, whereas others feel comfortable with the paternalistic doctor of old. Much also depends on how the patient feels at the time – their needs are not constant. June Huntington, who has contributed widely to management development in general practice, once said that she would complain just like any other 'customer' when kept waiting in out-patients, but that if she was feeling ill she 'reserved the right to behave like a patient'. It should also be remembered that the care which a doctor offers is different to that provided by a nurse.

General practitioners will continue to retain a degree of professional autonomy and status that is undreamed of by many other groups. With this they can largely manage their own time and work, in contrast to their hospital colleagues, they can act as advocates for their patients against the system, they can use their position in society for the benefit of the local community (being both part of the community and taking responsibility for it), and they may also possess a certain mystique which is linked to their perceived 'power over life and death'.

Finally, general practitioners exhibit a range of attributes and skills which are useful in any system of healthcare. They know how to consult with patients, and are trained in communication, clinical reasoning and problem solving. They are experienced in taking responsibility and making decisions, in general patients trust them, and they are used to working within the proper constraints of confidentiality. Above all, they are able to combine science with humanity, evidence-based medicine with personal care – *cum scientitia caritas* (as the motto of the Royal College of General Practitioners proclaims).

What do patients bring?

The wants of patients have been addressed in Chapter 11. But patients do not just bring demands and needs. They also bring the truth, at least the vast majority do. Many tell their general practitioners not only the truth about their lives as they see it, but also things about themselves which they would not divulge to anyone else. In doing so they confer on general practitioners an immense privilege, and their doctor becomes an important actor in their lives. For many patients their doctor walks down the road beside them as they endure their turbulent lives.

Patients also thank their doctors from time to time. Doctors who have moved out of clinical practice into management miss the immediate gratification of having a patient, once or twice a week, say to them: 'I feel better for having talked to you'.

Conclusion

The challenges are many, but the rewards (particularly the trust of patients) are significant. How often do we really seek patients' views? Box 13.5 shows the conclusions drawn from the study of Swedish diabetic patients.[23] There is clearly very real substance in the doctor–patient relationship, but the relationship does need both to enable and to accommodate dynamic change.

Box 13.5:   Patients' relationship with doctors

Patients are interested in:
- trust
- access
- partnership
- respect
- being seen as human
- quality of care.

Patients like doctors who:
- are easy to understand
- listen to the patient's story
- have knowledge about disease.

Patients:
- want to be part of the decision-making process
- are confident in their own expertise
- need education in order to understand different alternatives
- need high-quality information to enable them to make sensible choices.

But patients:
- fear scepticism among professionals
- worry about the use of outcome data (what is it used for?)
- are concerned about lack of time
- dread physician lack of interest.

Summary points

- General practice is being challenged from all quarters by consumerism, the threat of substitution, new demands for accountability, generational change and the 'new managerialism'.
- The forces behind these challenges are not all pulling in the same direction.
- Complexity theory provides a model for understanding the apparent chaos.
- Three 'rules' govern behaviour in the NHS, namely the needs to satisfy patients, professionals and government.
- None of the three is ever paramount and none is ever irrelevant.
- General practitioners will be involved in a number of functions of primary care, including consumer-responsive care, care based on a relationship, 'specialist' care and corporate governance.
- They will need to deploy a range of skills, and develop new skills in leadership and in working in partnership.
- There is real substance in the doctor–patient relationship.

References

1   Gray C (2000) Working on morale. *BMJ*. Classified Suppl. 8 July.

2   Theorell T (2000) Changing society: changing role of doctors. *BMJ*. **320**: 1417–18.

3   Coulter A (1999) Paternalism or partnership? Patients have grown up – and there's no going back. *BMJ*. **319**: 719–20.

4   Pereira Gray D (1998) Forty-seven minutes a year for the patient. *Br J Gen Pract*. **48**: 1816–17.

5   Social Exclusion Unit (1998) *Bringing Britain Together: a National Strategy for Neighbourhood Renewal*. Cabinet Office, London.

6   Statham D (2000) Guest editorial: partnership between health and social care. *Health Soc Care Commun*. **8**: 87–9.

7   Spencer J (1999) Educating the coming generation. In: T van Zwanenberg and J Harrison (eds) *Clinical Governance in Primary Care*. Radcliffe Medical Press, Oxford.

8   Hart JT (1988) *A New Kind of Doctor*. Merlin Press, London.

9   Department of Health (1986) *NHS Act 1977. Regulations*. HMSO, London.

10 British Medical Association (1965) *Charter for the Family Doctor Service*. British Medical Association, London.

11 Lewis J (1997) The changing meaning of the GP contract. *BMJ*. **314**: 895–8.

12 Hill P (1999) Reducing risk in primary care. In: T van Zwanenberg and J Harrison (eds) *Clinical Governance in Primary Care*. Radcliffe Medical Press, Oxford.

13 Taylor DH and Leese B (1997) Recruitment, retention, and time commitment change of general practitioners in England and Wales, 1990–4: a retrospective study. *BMJ*. **314**: 1806–10.

14 Harrison J (1998) Post-modern influences. In: J Harrison and T van Zwanenberg (eds) *GP Tomorrow*. Radcliffe Medical Press, Oxford.

15 Department of Health (2000) *The NHS Plan. A Plan for Investment. A Plan for Reform*. Department of Health, London; website (http://www.nhs.uk/nationalplan/htm)

16 Klein R and Dixon J (2000) Cash bonanza for NHS. The price is centralisation. *BMJ*. **320**: 883–4.

17 Beecham L (2000) Blair demands reform of the NHS. *BMJ*. **320**: 889.

18 Anon. (1935) The insurance medical service week by week: payment for keeping records. *BMJ*. **ii (Supplement)**: 174.

19 Anon. (2000) Editor's choice. The NHS: last act of a Greek tragedy? *BMJ*. **320**: 881.

20 Greenhalgh T (2000) Change and complexity – the rich picture. *Br J Gen Pract*. **50**: 514–15.

21 Kernick D (2000) Viewpoint. Plus ça change, plus c'est la meme chose. *Br J Gen Pract*. **50**: 591.

22 Department of Health (1998) *A Review of Continuing Professional Development in General Practice*. A Report by the Chief Medical Officer. Department of Health, London.

23 Fallberg L (2000) Can patients make 'sensible' choices in health care? A Nordic perspective. European Health Management Association Conference, Orebro, Sweden. 29 June 2000.

24 van Zwanenberg T (1998) GP tomorrow. In: J Harrison and T van Zwanenberg (eds) *GP Tomorrow*. Radcliffe Medical Press, Oxford.

25 Calman K (1998) Lessons from Whitehall. *BMJ*. **317**: 1718–20.

26 Koeck C (1998) Time for organisational development in healthcare organisations. *BMJ*. **317**: 1267–8.

27 Purves I (1998) The changing consultation. In: J Harrison and T van Zwanenberg (eds) *GP Tomorrow*. Radcliffe Medical Press, Oxford.

CHAPTER FOURTEEN

Conclusion – the future and the new GP

Jamie Harrison

There is a place again for that kind of generalist, someone who can wander among special-ised fields and pull things together. Otherwise it's very compartmentalised and syntheses don't really happen.

Bob Brain on Bruce Chatwin

This final chapter draws together key strands from the book and considers three modes of being for the new GP.

Although it is impossible to judge how long the current New Labour government will last, there is no doubt that much of the modernisation programme that has been set in motion will survive. Whatever the shape or character of what follows, themes of quality improvement, greater accountability, value for money and improved performance will remain. Moreover, the medical profession will need to be increasingly responsive to the concerns and expectations of patients and politicians alike if it is to maintain its high social standing and relative freedom from external regulation. But how should the new GP seek to maintain personal and professional integrity in such a changing world?

The generalist

The above quotation from Nicholas Shakespeare's biography of the author and adventurer Bruce Chatwin reminds us of one of his particular qualities. Chatwin saw through the surface to the deeper issues within a culture or society, expressing such insights with clarity and sophistication. This gift did not always win him friends. He had a broad approach, with expertise in the world of art, archaeology and literature. He was a true generalist – one who could 'pull things together'.

In our increasingly fragmented, postmodern world, the gift of synthesis – of being able to see the bigger picture and hold issues in tension – is ever more necessary. Patients come to their doctor with many different needs at different times and places in their lives. Often they feel ill-equipped to make decisions, either because they lack the necessary information or because their illness hinders their capacity to make effective decisions. The clinical judgement of the doctor, in empathetic relationship with the patient, still counts for a lot.

The new GPs will also be asked to comment on and take decisions about the wider provision of health services – as those actively involved in commissioning services within the context of a PCG or a PCT. In addition, they will be providers of more specialised services within their own GP practices, as more of the traditional secondary care activity is transferred to primary care. They would therefore do well to remember their generalist roots – their heritage as 'someone who can wander amongst specialised fields and pull things together'.

The mediator

Mediation is the art of reconciling, of making connections and links, and of bringing together what is separated. The above-noted fragmentation in society is mirrored by fragmentation in the health service at every level. GP partnerships and practice teams are all too often dysfunctional – disunited and pulling in opposing directions – even though the majority of individuals concerned are dedicated and able clinicians, wanting to do their best. The newly evolving PCGs and PCTs face the same issues. There is a place for those who mediate and negotiate to make meaningful and lasting peace.

Mediators are also those who lead by example, setting aside personal agendas and professional preferences to find a positive way forward. However, that does not involve making soft decisions, fudging the issue or accepting weak compromises. Good mediation should lead to strong outcomes and clear benefits to all.

The way of mediation resonates with enduring GP roles – of being both gatekeeper to the health services and advocate of the patient, not least in an age of resource 'rationing' and consumer pressure. The gatekeeper must inevitably keep one eye on the available resources and how best to utilise them. The other eye needs to focus on the patient in the consultation – the immediate need that requires an answer. The mediator must make the links, clarify the issues and draw together what is separated, not least linking between the proper demands of the patient and the wider world of the NHS.

The covenanter

A covenanter is someone who enters voluntarily into relationships with others based on trust and mutuality. Covenanting is risky in that trust can be misplaced or betrayed. Recent events highlighted in the media have undermined the trust between doctor and patient.

However, much within the central section of this book seeks to encourage a new covenant between doctor, patient and society. A greater openness, allied to the willingness to embrace continuing professional development, revalidation and appraisal, is to be welcomed – not least as a means of starting to rebuild bridges with the public. And public confidence can only be fully restored when access to healthcare is fair and equitable, robust quality mechanisms are in place, and healthcare professionals working in effective teams are the norm. Doctor and patient can then face the outside world united.

To be a covenanter also requires a willingness to say 'no' when the pressure is too great, for to respond unthinkingly to every demand (however worthy) does not benefit either doctors or patients. Such a robust response may be controversial within our medical culture, but it remains a key component of covenantal relationships, which are for the good of all.

Conclusion

Fulfilling this vision for the new GP requires professional confidence, courage and the willingness to take risks. Members of the new breed of doctors will not slavishly follow their predecessors. They will demand a good working environment, decent pay and conditions, and a say in how the organisation is run. Yet the challenge to them will be to engage with the broader perspective of having both the privilege and responsibility of being a GP. Their medical training should equip them as technicians and communicators, and make them empathetic and aware of patient needs. They will also begin to learn about managing public health through PCTs. Ultimately, however, they must decide for themselves how and whether to embrace the three modes outlined above. The future of general practice depends on their decision, and for its part the NHS will need to provide the new GP with the necessary space and support.

Index

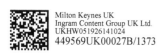

Milton Keynes UK
Ingram Content Group UK Ltd.
UKHW051926141024
449569UK00027B/1373